CANADIAN MEDICAL LIVES

WILLIAM R. BEAUMONT
Mechanical Genius

by Julian A. Smith
Series Editor: T.P. Morley

Associated Medical Services, Incorporated
&
Fitzhenry & Whiteside
1995

Copyright© Associated Medical Services Incorporated/The Hannah Institute for the History of Medicine, 1995

Fitzhenry & Whiteside
195 Allstate Parkway
Markham, Ontario L3R 4T8

All rights reserved. No part of this publication may be reproduced, stored in a retrieval system, or transmitted in any form or by any means, electronic, mechanical, photocopying, recording, or otherwise, except brief passages for purposes of review, without the prior permission of Fitzhenry & Whiteside.

Jacket design: Arne Roosman
Copy Editor: Nicholas Stephens
Typesetting: Cortland Design
Printing and Binding: Gagné Printing Ltd., Louiseville, Quebec, Canada

Fitzhenry & Whiteside wishes to acknowledge the generous assistance and ongoing support of **The Book Publishing Industry Development Programme of the Department of Communications, The Canada Council, and The Ontario Arts Council.**

Care has been taken to trace the ownership of copyright material used in the text, including the illustrations. The author and publisher welcome any information enabling them to rectify any reference or credit in subsequent editions.

Canadian Cataloguing In Publication Data

Smith, Julian (Julian A.)
    William R. Beaumont, mechanical genius

(Canadian medical lives ; no. 10)
Co-published by the Hannah Institute for the History of Medicine.
Includes bibliographical references and index.
ISBN 1-55041-159-4

1. Beaumont, William R., 1803-1875. 2. Surgical instruments and apparatus – Canada – History – 19th century. 3. Surgeons – Canada – Biography. 4. Inventors – Canada – Biography. I. Hannah Institute for the History of Medicine. II. Title. III. series.

RD27.35.B43S55 1994   617'.092   C94-932801-4

CANADIAN MEDICAL LIVES SERIES

The Story of the Hannah Institute for the History of Medicine has been told by John B. Neilson and G.R. Paterson in *Associated Medical Services Incorporated: A History* (1987). Dr. Donald R. Wilson, President of AMS, and the Board of directors decided that the Institute should produce this series of biographies as one of its undertakings.

The first ten biographies can be obtained through the retail book trade, or from Dundurn Press Ltd., 2181 Queen Street East, Suite 301, Toronto, ON M4E 1E3, and Dundurn Distribution, 73 Lime Walk, Headington, Oxford, England 0X3 7AD.

The second group of biographies, of which this is the seventh volume, can also be obtained through retail book stores, or from Fitzhenry & Whiteside, 195 Allstate Parkway, Markham, ON L3R 4T8.

In the annals of Canadian medicine, William Beaumont has attracted attention through his alleged unwitting contribution to Singer's invention of the sewing machine. As Julian Smith shows, there is little or no support for the claim, nor does Beaumont need such conspicuous attention to establish himself as an important figure in surgery and medical teaching in the first half of the nineteenth century.

T.P. Morley
Series Editor
1995

CANADIAN MEDICAL LIVES SERIES

Dundurn Press:

Duncan Graham by Robert Kerr and Douglas Waugh

Bill Mustard by Marilyn Dunlop

Joe Doupe by Terence Moore

Clarence Hincks by Charles G. Roland

Francis Scrimger by Suzanne Kingsmill

Emily Stowe by Mary Beacock Fryer

R.G. Ferguson by C. Stuart Houston

Harold Griffith by Richard Bodman and Deirdre Gillies

Earle P. Scarlett by F.W. Musselwhite

Maude Abbott by Douglas Waugh

Fitzhenry & Whiteside:

William Boyd by Ian Carr

J.C. Boileau Grant by C.L.N. Robinson

R.M. Bucke by Peter A. Rechnitzer

William Henry Drummond by J.B. Lyons

Alan Brown by A.B. Kingsmill

Harold N. Segall by C.G. Roland

William R. Beaumont by Julian A. Smith

CONTENTS

List of illustrations 8
Acknowledgements 9
Prologue 11
  1.   The Early Years 15
  2.   Surgeon and Inventor 30
  3.   The Toronto Medical Community 48
  4.   Lectures Composed with Great Care 58
  5.   Surgeon and Administrator 66
  6.   Scandals, Scholars and Sclerotica 80
  7.   Medical Schools at War 91
  8.   The Profession Is Indebted 98
  9.   He should have Dr. Beaumont 109
10.   New Hospitals and New Surgeons 121
11.   Army Surgeon at Last 133
12.   Did Beaumont Invent the Sewing Machine? 141
13.   Conclusion 153
       Bibliography 157
       Notes and References 173
       Index 185

To my parents
Dr. Robert S. Smith and Mrs. Dorian Smith

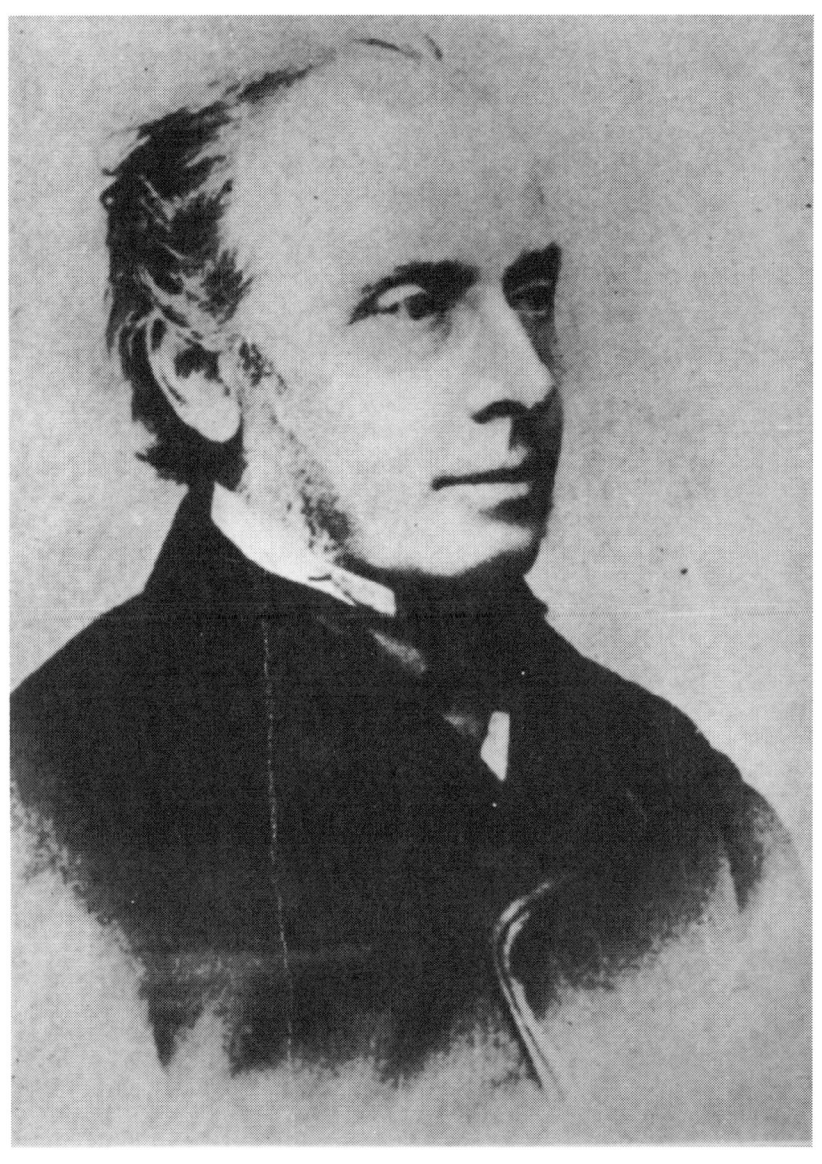

William Rawlins Beaumont. *From a painting in the Academy of Medicine, Toronto*

LIST OF ILLUSTRATIONS

1. William Rawlins Beaumont. (From a painting in the Academy of Medicine.)
2. St. Bartholomew's Hospital Quadrangle, 1830. (Roberts, 1989, 39.)
3. York (Toronto) General Hospital, 1820. (Robertson, Landmarks of Toronto, Vol. 1, 1913.)
4. King's College Medical School, 1844. (Godfrey, 112.)
5. Toronto General Hospital, 1854–1878. (Spragge.)
6. Trinity College Medical School, 1871. (Canada Lancet, Sept. 1871).
7. Toronto General Hospital, 1913.
8. Rocket shaft, 1862. (Beaumont, Lancet, June 14, 1862.)
9. Fistulae instrument, 1836. (Beaumont, Medico–Chirurgical Transactions, 21, 1838).
10. Speculum vaginae, 1836. (Beaumont, London Medical Gazette, April 27, 1837.)
11. Deep suturing instrument, 1837. (Bell's Sketch, 1976. Original in the Toronto Museum of History of Medicine.)
12. Iris forceps, 1863. (Beaumont, "New Iris Forceps," 176.)
13. Fixation forceps. (Down Brothers., 1901.)
14. Canalicula knife. (Tiemann, 1889, 148.)
15. Fracture instrument, 1851. (Beaumont, Upper Canada Journal of Medical, Surgical and Physical Science, 2, 1852–53, 157–158.)
16. How the legend began. ("Medical News: The Sewing Machine," Lancet, March 17, 1866.)
17. Elias Howe's Original Machine, 1846. (Chisholm, 744.)
18. Isaac Singer's Original Machine, 1851. (Chisholm, 744.)
19. Beaumont's goods at death, 1875. (Archives of Ontario.)
20. Beaumont's Will. (Archives of Ontario.)

Acknowledgements

This book owes a great debt to many people and institutions. It would not have been written at all were it not for the encouragement and support of Pauline Mazumdar, Professor of the History of Medicine at the Institute for the History and Philosophy of Science and Technology at Victoria College in the University of Toronto.

The research has been carried out largely in and around Toronto. Its many libraries and archives have been constant sources of information. Foremost on the list are those of the University of Toronto. The Science and Medicine Library and the John P. Robarts Research Library were very helpful, particularly through the Thomas Fisher Rare Book Room, the Government Documents Section, and the Microfilm Department. From these sources it was possible to research Beaumont's days at King's College and his administrative life in the 1850s and 1860s. Henri Pilon probed the Trinity College Archives for information on Beaumont's work there in the 1870s. Pilon and his colleagues, especially David Roberts and Monica Sandor, graciously made the extensive library and archives of the *Dictionary of Canadian Biography* at 243 College Street available to me. The staff of the Baldwin Room at the Metro Toronto Reference Library at 789 Yonge Street found several useful Beaumont items.

The staff at St. James's Cathedral Archives at 131 Adelaide Street East helped me find baptismal, marriage and burial records for Beaumont's immediate family. Important death records were also kindly made available by St. James Cemetery at 635 Parliament Street. The staff at the library of the Ontario Genealogical Society in the North York Public Library at 5120 Yonge Street unearthed Beaumont's English roots. The extensive

Genealogical Library of the Church of Jesus Christ of Latter Day Saints (Mormons) at 95 Melbert Street in Etobicoke was also helpful in tracing members of the Beaumont family.

A major source of biographical material on Beaumont is to be found in the Archives of Ontario at 77 Grenville Street. I gratefully acknowledge the staff's providing me with census records, the Strachan Papers, the Canniff Papers, rare Canadian medical journals, various marriage records and Beaumont's Will. Equally helpful was the staff at the Archives of the City of Toronto in Nathan Phillips Square, where I was guided through countless York and Toronto City Assessment Rolls, Directories, local histories and other documents. The staff also helped me on the background of Beaumont's financial circumstances.

For information about 19th century surgical instruments, including Beaumont's, one can do no better than to consult the library and the museum of the Toronto Academy of Medicine, now at the Toronto General Hospital. Beaumont's deep-suturing instrument and many rare surgical instrument catalogues from the 19th century are all to be found there.

Finally, I would like to thank Alison Li and Michelle Jugandi, who read and improved the manuscript at several stages of its evolution. Their indefatigable support was always helpful, although the responsibility for any errors is of course mine alone.

Julian A. Smith,
Toronto.

Prologue

It was a warm Wednesday evening in the spring of 1859 and the Irish insurgent William Smith O'Brien was preparing to face a crowd. Three thousand people had gathered in front of the Rossin House in downtown Toronto to hear him speak about his violent efforts to overthrow British rule in Ireland, including his important work as leader of the abortive 1848 uprising in County Tipperary. For his part in this insurrection he was at first sentenced to death, but his punishment was later commuted to deportation to Van Diemen's Land. By 1856 his exemplary conduct had earned him a full pardon from the British government. O'Brien was now free to embark on a tour of North America to meet the thousands of Irish exiles who had flocked to the United States and Canada seeking freedom and employment.

Now here he was in Toronto, and the city's Irish were out in force. They loudly applauded his tales of courage, resistance and freedom. Musicians played Irish songs and patriots shot fireworks into the air. It was truly a festive atmosphere and the crowd was ready to celebrate all night.

At the nearby Toronto General Hospital on Gerrard Street East, Dr. William Rawlins Beaumont had been tramping the wards all day, seeing patients in the morning, teaching medical students in the afternoon and helping other doctors with their more difficult operations. And then he had had to attend to his own private patients. Perhaps he could rest over a glass of wine with his friend, Doctor Edward Hodder.

Suddenly, a frightened man burst in on him.

"Doctor Beaumont," he cried, "come quick! There's been an accident at O'Brien's speech!"

The doctor followed the man to the nearby Shakespeare Tavern at the corner of York and King Streets. Pushing his way through the crowd of spectators, he reached the bar where James Watkins, a tall, lean, middle-aged man was slumped motionless in a chair, his countenance pale with shock. A splinter of wood was sticking out of his face between his nose and left eye. His features were pallid and shrunken.

"What happened?" Beaumont asked.

"He got hit by a rocket," the man explained. "We were firing them and he got hit just a few minutes ago! He walked in here and sat down and I ran to get you."

"He walked in here? By himself? Through that crowd?" Beaumont could hardly believe it.

Celebrants had been shooting off fireworks all evening long. One carelessly fired rocket had run off horizontally into the crowd. It went straight through a man's hat and then struck Watkins in the face at a distance of only 11 metres. He had walked about 30 metres to the tavern, where he had collapsed into a chair.

Beaumont laid him down on the floor, propped up his head and shoulders and set to work. Judging by the length of the protruding stick, he guessed the rocket must have penetrated at least 15 centimetres into the man's head. Strangely, though, there was no blood![1]

As Beaumont examined Watkins, some of the crowd outside came into the tavern and, curious and fearful, watched him operate on the luckless victim. "James doesn't have a chance," his friends lamented in hushed voices. "But this is no ordinary doctor," others murmured. "This is the great Beaumont! He's the best surgeon in the whole city; if there's anyone who can save Watkins, it's him!"

Beaumont took his strongest forceps from his bag and pulled at the splinter. It wouldn't budge. He sent for a pair of pliers from Mr. Grainger's business nearby, but the rocket was wedged tight. He could rotate it a little, but it would not come out. Just how deep was the thing buried, anyway? And if he did manage to get it out, what then?

Injuries of this type were almost always fatal, Beaumont thought to himself. After all, hadn't his old teacher back in medical school, the great doctor John Abernethy, said as much? But Abernethy had never had modern tools at his disposal!

Beaumont was probably the best equipped doctor in Toronto. He had made quite a name for himself already by inventing many surgical instruments, from an iris forceps to a vaginal speculum. And then there was the tool he had invented some 20 years ago to stitch up deep wounds. Local people were even saying that this instrument had inspired the fabulously successful Singer sewing machine! Who was this inventor-surgeon? Did he really invent the principle of the sewing machine? And what was he doing in Upper Canada?

* * * *

William Rawlins Beaumont (1803-1875) was a surgeon equally at home in the workshop and the hospital who balanced the competing demands of government, administration and university teaching and who impressed a generation of Canadian doctors with his zeal, charity and ability. To no less a doctor than William Osler he was "the highest type of the cultivated English surgeon." Osler told his students that in Beaumont they could finally see "the leaven which has raised our profession above the dead level of a business."[2]

Beaumont stood on the threshold of an era that was to enthusiastically embrace science and technology, and that was to hold sacred the ideal of progress through invention and engineering. The nineteenth century saw a flurry of scientific advances in European and American workshops. There were great developments in a variety of medical instruments, ranging all the way from simple knives to complex microscopes.

For example, the first true achromatic microscopes — the Universal models of the French and Italian designers Chevalier and Amici — belonged to the 1820s. The English surgeon Robert Liston (1794-1847) popularized the long straight-bladed amputation knife in the 1840s. And James Marion Sims (1813-1883) in New York designed the famous vaginal speculum around 1845. Surgical forceps were radically improved throughout this era too, culminating in the incorporation of a locking device by Sir Thomas Spencer Wells (1818-1897). Meanwhile, Arthur Learned presented an early binaural stethoscope in 1851 to the London International Exhibition. The 1850s also saw the double-bladed pocket scalpel and the easily sterilized all-metal scalpel was well in vogue by 1880. All over the world new instruments were revolutionizing the practice of surgery.[3]

Furthermore, the introduction of anaesthesia and antiseptics in medicine was overturning centuries of surgical practice. Before the 1840s, surgery had depended more on speed than accuracy. Amputations typically took only a few minutes and demanded nerves of steel and a studied deafness to a patient's heartrending cries of pain. By the 1840s, several new anesthetics at last allowed relatively pain-free operations. In 1842 the American surgeon Crawford Williamson Long (1815-1878) used ether for minor operations and by 1844 it was being used in dentistry by Horace Wells (1815-1848). In 1847 chloroform was successfully introduced into surgery by the Scottish obstetrician James Young Simpson (1811-1870).

Now at last the surgeon could take his time over his operations.[4]

Antiseptics followed shortly afterwards. Before the 1860s, many patients who had successfully undergone surgery died later from infection. No modern advances in surgery were possible until sepsis had been conquered. The pioneer in the application of Pasteur's microbial theory to clinical surgery was Joseph Lister (1827-1912), who introduced, around 1867, carbolic acid into the operating room. This affected a profound change in surgical practice and finally made internal operations safe and therefore practical.[5]

Surgical practice altered so radically during the 40-year period from 1830 to 1870 that earlier teachers of medicine could scarcely have imagined the changes their students would see. Beaumont was in the forefront of all these innovations. He kept abreast of surgical developments in Europe and America and was among the first to introduce chloroform, new surgical instruments and clean dressings to Canada.

Beaumont's role in the invention of surgical tools is probably what he is best known for. He has been called "a prolific inventor of surgical instruments,"[6] and virtually all sources agree he was a very capable surgeon to boot.[7] Donald Jack has gone so far as to call him the true "father of surgical instruments in Upper Canada."[8] However, despite these accolades, precise information about his role in developing medical instruments has so far been unavailable.[9]

Beaumont's work in Canada coincided with several important events in Toronto medical history. He saw the founding of King's College, the Toronto School of Medicine and Trinity University, and ended up working for them all. He trained a new generation of famous Canadian doctors, including Osler, Aikins and Canniff. He took an active part in early efforts to raise professional standards in medicine. Moreover, he encouraged the rapid proliferation of hospitals in Toronto and approved the increased role of government in Canadian medical practice.

This book records the remarkable life of an inventor-physician whom University of Toronto anatomy professor James Richardson later called "the ideal of a surgeon."

—— Chapter 1 ——

Irish Emigrants

William Rawlins Beaumont was born on tiny Beaumont Street in Marylebone, London, England, in September 1803. Marylebone is a district in London's West End, now sandwiched between Regent's Park and Hyde Park. It got its name from the Church of St. Mary's by the Bourne, built around 1400 in an effort to renovate and revitalize the disreputable and violent neighbourhood of Tyburn.

William was baptized in the Anglican Church of St. Marylebone, on St. Marylebone Road in the parish of St. Mary's. His parents, Edward and Charlotte Beaumont, were part of a family that had come from France and settled in England at the beginning of the 14th century.[10]

William spent his childhood under the watchful eye of his elder brother, Edward Beaumont (1801-?). As far as we know, there were no other children in the Beaumont house. Six years earlier, Charlotte had given birth to a daughter, Ann, who died in infancy. So William and Edward grew up on their own and soon learned to look out for each other in the rough and tumble world of early nineteenth century London. They forged a friendship that would survive William's move to Canada; 50 years later, Edward would travel to Toronto to visit William and sponsor his son Herbert for baptism.

Beaumont Street had been laid out in 1778 across Marylebone Gardens, which the *Daily Courant* had considered "much the pleasantest place about town...and thought by the nobility and gentry to be very commodious for breakfast." When the proprietor's lease expired in 1777, the garden was subdivided into plots by Sir Beaumont Hotham and leased to builders. Soon it was full of various branches of the Beaumont family. Edward and Charlotte occupied one of the newly constructed homes. When William was born, there was still plenty of open space for a young boy to play, but urban development soon pressed north against the New Road (Marylebone Road), and Beaumont Street became quite congested. Fortunately for William, Regent's Park was developed nearby and he once again had lots of room.

The street where William grew up is now largely commercial, with medical offices and retail shops. The King Edward VII Hospital for Officers takes up the eastern side and on the west stand Waverley Court, Beaumont Court and the hospital's Nurses' Home. The park, of course, is still there, but today it includes the famous London Zoo and Queen Mary Gardens.

Beaumont received a sound, liberal education in several private schools in London,[11] but not much is known of this period in his life. He began his medical studies at an early age as a student in St. Bartholomew's Hospital across town.

St. Bartholomew's was founded in 1123 by a monk named Rahere (?-1144) who, after surviving a bout of malaria during a pilgrimage to Rome, vowed to create a refuge for London's sick and destitute. Saint Bartholomew appeared in a vision to him and told him to build the hospital on the swampy executioner's ground at Smithfield which, when cleared, proved to be so well adapted to his design that today's Hospital of St. Bartholomew still stands on Rahere's original site.

The hospital was made up of clusters of buildings around several courtyards to provide a sheltered environment for the inmates and promote a feeling of community. It was later run by the Austin Canons, members of a well-known Augustinian monastery, who, with a small group of nearby nuns, cared for the sick, took in and educated orphans and sheltered the homeless. Over the years the hospital became quite an important force in the City of London and was well provided with funds and properties from rich benefactors. It was given a royal charter by Henry VIII, which guaranteed it support from the City of London and placed its management in lay hands.

William Harvey (1578-1657) was appointed physician to St. Bartholomew's in 1609.[12] In 1628 he published *Exercitatio Anatomica de Motu Cordis et Sanguinis in Animalibus*, "the most important medical work ever written." The hospital survived the Civil War, the outbreak of plague in 1665 and the Great Fire of London in 1666, although several nearby shops and houses were destroyed. The early eighteenth century saw the beginning of a rebuilding programme by the architect James Gibbs (1682-1754), who restored the hospital's original courtyard design, creating four surrounding wings of three storeys each. The buildings were completed in 1769.

The hospital's medical school, which Beaumont attended, dated back to the seventeenth century, when young doctors accompanied senior physicians during their ward rounds. A museum for surgical and anatomical specimens was opened in 1726, and in 1767 doctors were allowed to use the operating theatre and a nearby room as lecture halls. Percival Pott (1713-1788), one of the great surgeons of the period, was apprenticed at the hospital in 1729 and was among the first to teach in these classrooms. However, it was the celebrated surgeon and teacher John Abernethy (1764-1831) who formally founded the medical school.

Abernethy had a lasting influence on the young Beaumont. He had been an assistant surgeon at St. Bartholomew's since 1787, and had begun lecturing there soon after. He was appointed assistant surgeon to Christ's Hospital in 1813, and the following year Professor of Anatomy and Surgery at the College of Surgeons. Over the next decade he gained a wide reputation for his daring but careful operations for the cure of aneurysm. His teachings on this subject were later to be of value to Beaumont. Abernethy published several surgical texts and laid down two medical principles that greatly influenced later surgical practice: that local disease had a constitutional origin, and that this origin could usually be traced to disorders of the digestive system.[13]

It was through his brilliance as a lecturer that Abernethy first met the young Beaumont. Abernethy lectured on anatomy, physiology and surgery. As his classes became more crowded, he successfully petitioned the hospital's House Committee to construct an expanded lecture theatre. Over 400 attended his first lecture in the new theatre on 1 October 1822.

"The theatre was crowded to its capacity on the day Abernethy was to lecture. He never entered the place without being cheered, the applause rising and dying away the instant he began to speak...always something new and worth listening to, and delivered in his own inimitable and vigorous style."[14]

Would that more of today's medical lecturers were so popular with their students!

Abernethy was evidently quite impressed with the young Beaumont. He quickly appointed him his medical dresser, and the two formed a strong bond that lasted until Abernethy's death in 1831. Late in his life, Abernethy fondly recalled Beaumont as a student who "did very assiduously prosecute his professional studies at St. Bartholomew's Hospital for more than an ordinary length of time."[15]

Beaumont was equally impressed with Abernethy. He particularly liked his mentor's lecturing style. Abernethy was fond of repeating little anecdotes to illustrate the complicated medical information he was trying to impart. One of his stories made a deep impression on Beaumont.

Two children were playing together, and one went into another room and closed the door. When the second child put his eye to the keyhole, the first pushed a small stick into the poor boy's eye. The boy died from the wound to the brain, even though the force of the thrust had been very small. Beaumont remembered this story all his life, and was to use it almost 40 years later in his lectures after one of his own patients survived a more brutal attack.[16]

Beaumont quickly saw that success at the medical school depended very much on self-discipline. Students were largely left to themselves. They registered for and attended lectures at the hospital on their own initiative and had little guidance. Some industrious students attended lectures at several different hospitals while a number of "grinding schools," such as the nearby Aldersgate Street School, offered lectures and demonstrations by famous teachers outside the hospitals altogether. It was largely up to the student to find out what classes were available and to seek them out. But if it was impossible to attend a certain doctor's lectures, a student need not despair. Several of the most celebrated physicians, including Abernethy, published their lectures in *The Lancet*, founded in 1823 by Thomas Wakley (1795-1882), the London surgeon. Beaumont later published several of his own clinical lectures in the same journal.

Some medical students of Beaumont's day worked quite hard at their studies; others were lazy, indifferent or incompetent. They had a reputation for being immoral, vulgar in speech and coarse in behaviour. One of them, Sir James Paget (1814-1899), who entered St. Bartholomew's about a decade later than Beaumont, recalled his colleagues in these terms: "As for the general body of the students of my time, I believe they were, in comparison with others of the same age and same level, about as they are now... As among other students, there were a few thoroughly vicious fellows who came to a bad end, left the school in disgrace, or were plucked and not heard of more; and some idle fools; and some blockheads and untaught, who could never learn their duty. These have been caricatured as if they were types of the whole class; it would be as reasonable to sketch the general character of Englishmen from a slight acquaintance with some inmates of an insane asylum. The majority of students then, as now, worked well; some were laborious, as with a natural pleasure in the exercise of mental power, or in emulation, or in consciousness of duty or of necessity, or with all these motives."[17]

If the majority of Beaumont's fellow students worked hard, they played even harder. As Paget explains: "There is a greater contrast in the play than in the work of that time than this. The pleasures and amusements then were coarser. There was much more drinking; a few were often drunk, and many who never were so would boast of drinking more than they thought they needed. Cursing and swearing were common in ordinary talk, frequent for emphasis, and nasty stories were very often told and deemed of the same worth as witty ones. Impurity of life and conversation were scarcely thought disgraceful or worth concealing. But in all these faults there were great differences among the students; some might boast of them, but many only tolerated them and kept as clear as they could; a few rebuked them, chiefly those who, in the slang of those days, were called saints or Simeonites, after the great Cambridge preacher."[18] It would be wrong to blame the students entirely for their failings. Many were following the examples set for them by their teachers. Some of their lecturers often used coarse language and bawdy mnemonics in their classes to help their students remember lists of facts.

Beaumont's position as dresser under Abernethy before his retirement in 1827 gave him the opportunity to see many unusual medical problems on which to practise his rapidly developing surgical skills. One particularly difficult case was that of the unfortunate John Turner.

John Turner, a boy of about eight or nine, had been accidentally run over in the street by the wheel of a cart. He was brought to St. Bartholomew's Hospital about eight o'clock in the evening on 25 August 1825, where he was placed under Beaumont's care. Beaumont's poignant description of the child reveal his efforts to revive him. "He breathed with extreme difficulty, seemingly by the diaphragm and abdominal muscles alone; he was restless, his pulse small and feeble, and his limbs, I thought, were colder than the ordinary temperature of one's body. Between 20 and 30 leeches were applied to his chest."[19]

Beaumont then allowed his patient to rest. A few hours later, "The neck and left side of the thorax became emphysematous; but on the right side there was scarcely any emphysema. I put on the rib bandage, which at first afforded relief, but the emphysema increasing, and the patient complaining the bandage was painful, I removed it." Yet Turner continued to deteriorate. "About one o'clock, the difficulty of breathing had become so great that every inspiration seemed to be the patient's last." At this point Beaumont decided that drastic measures were necessary and he began to operate on the child. The notes he made that night describe the operation:

"An opening was now made into the left cavity of the thorax, in the situation where the emphysema was first observed, and where it existed to the greatest extent. Immediately, on the pleura (costalis) being divided, there followed a sound as of air rushing through the wound, and in about five minutes the patient died."

He decided to carry out a post mortem examination. He found to his surprise that the left side of the chest, which had supposedly received the greatest injury, in fact showed the least; the collapsed lung was bruised in only a few places, and "the pleura seemed lacerated." The right side, however, showed substantially more damage: there was one fractured rib, a more severely collapsed lung, and "there penetrated deep into its substance an excessive wound...which must have been enormous before the lung collapsed." Further investigation led him to conclude that "the whole of the bones and cartilage yielded so far as to allow one of the ribs (and most likely that which was fractured, which, having only its cartilaginous attachment to the sternum, would yield the most) to be pressed with such force against the lung as to make, blunt as it is, the wound I have described."[20] In other words, the injury to the lung had actually been caused by the fractured rib, not the cartwheel alone.

While studying and working at St. Bartholomew's, Beaumont cultivated friendships with several other important doctors. One of these was Sir Astley Paston Cooper (1768-1841), who was later to become President of the Royal College of Surgeons (1827) and Vice-President of the Royal Society (1830). Educated in Edinburgh, Cooper had become a demonstrator of anatomy at St. Thomas's Hospital in London in 1789. By 1800 he had become surgeon to London's Guy's Hospital. His great work, *The Anatomy* and *Surgical Treatment of Hernia*, was already published when Beaumont began his studies under him. Cooper was created baronet in 1820 after removing a small tumour from the head of King George IV. He pioneered in the surgery of blood vessels, experimental surgery and in the surgery of the ear, and was said to have dissected on every day of his working life.[21]

Beaumont also studied neurology under Herbert Mayo (1796-1852) during this time. Mayo practised surgery and taught anatomy in London between 1819 and 1843; he also became surgeon to the Middlesex Hospital and founded the medical school there in 1836. In *Anatomical and Physiological Commentaries*, he recognized the sensory function of the fifth cranial nerve and the motor function of the seventh (facial) nerve.[22] This important research into the physiology of nerves was conducted independently of similar work by Charles Bell (1774-1842) and François Magendie (1783-1855).[23]

Another of Beaumont's teachers was the anatomist and physiologist Sir William Lawrence (1783-1867), who had been apprenticed to Abernethy at St. Bartholomew's Hospital in 1799, later replacing him as surgical lecturer. Much of Lawrence's career was tied to this hospital. He had already been a demonstrator before his appointment as surgeon to the hospital in 1824, a position he held until his retirement in 1865. Lawrence became notorious for his lectures criticizing Abernethy's defence of vitalism, as well as his argument that all mental activities were merely functions of the brain, rather than reflecting an immortal soul or spirit.[24] Theologians of the day considered this sort of reasoning to be perilously close to atheism, and rebuked him sharply. But while these claims made Lawrence famous, he is more important in the Beaumont story for his work in ophthalmology.

Lawrence was one of the most distinguished eye surgeons of the early 19th century.[25] He was surgeon to the London Infirmary for Curing Diseases of the Eye. Beaumont probably acquired most of his knowledge of ophthalmology from Lawrence, which he put to good use when he moved to Canada, where he designed several ophthalmological instruments based on those of Lawrence, and where he carried out extensive eye surgery.

Lawrence's classes, which Beaumont attended, were quite well received. Paget, one of Beaumont's later friends, considered them among the most important contributions to his studies. He said the lectures "...of Lawrence were, I think, the best then given in London: admirable in their

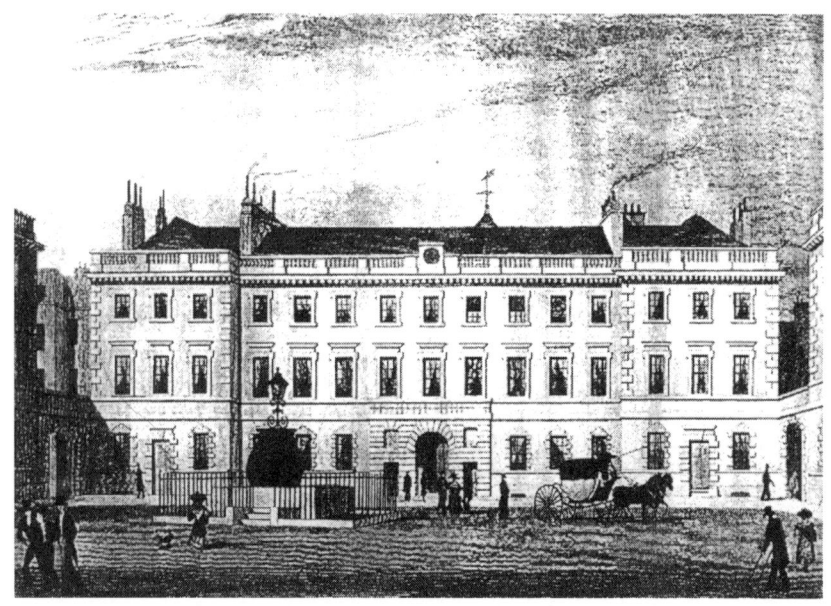

St. Bartholomew's Hospital Quadrangle, 1830. (Roberts, 1989, 39.)

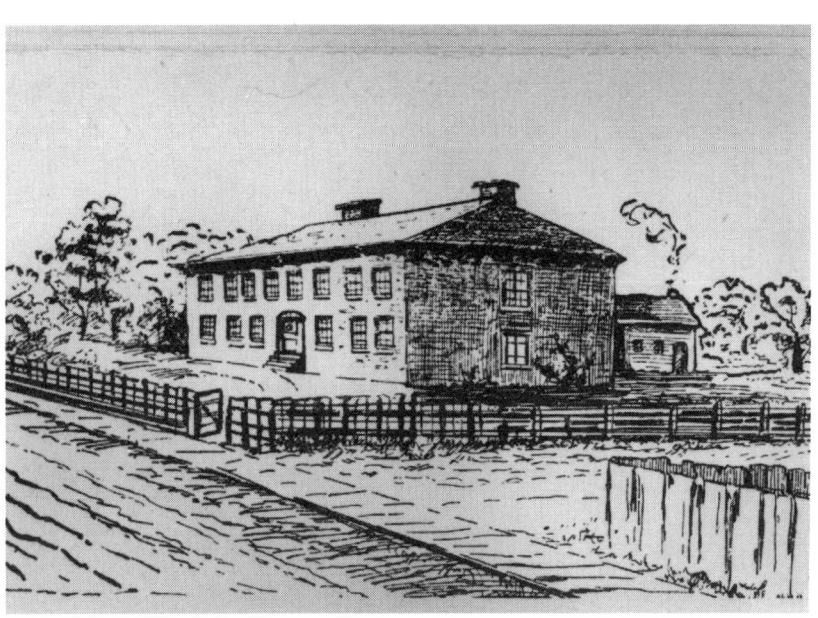

York (Toronto) General Hospital, 1820. (Robertson, Landmarks of Toronto, Vol. 1, 1913

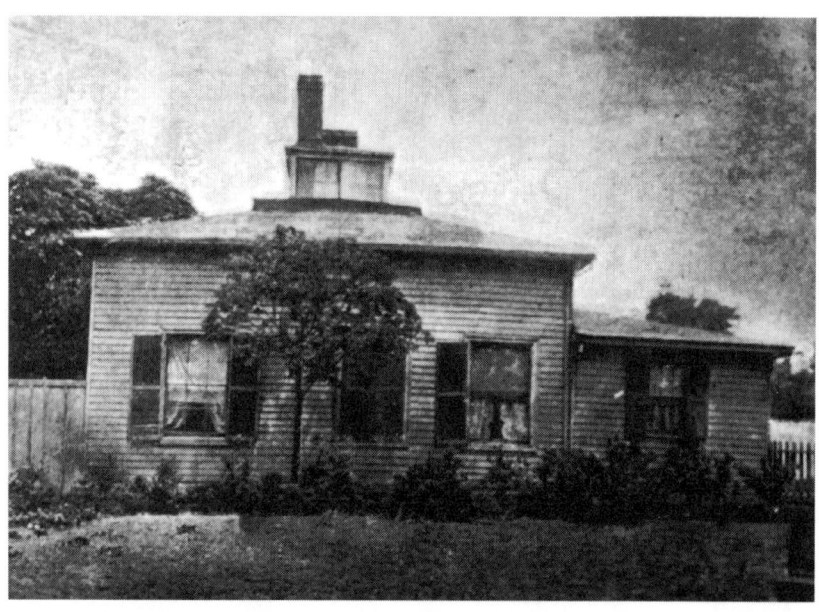

King's College Medical School, 1844. (Godfrey, 112.)

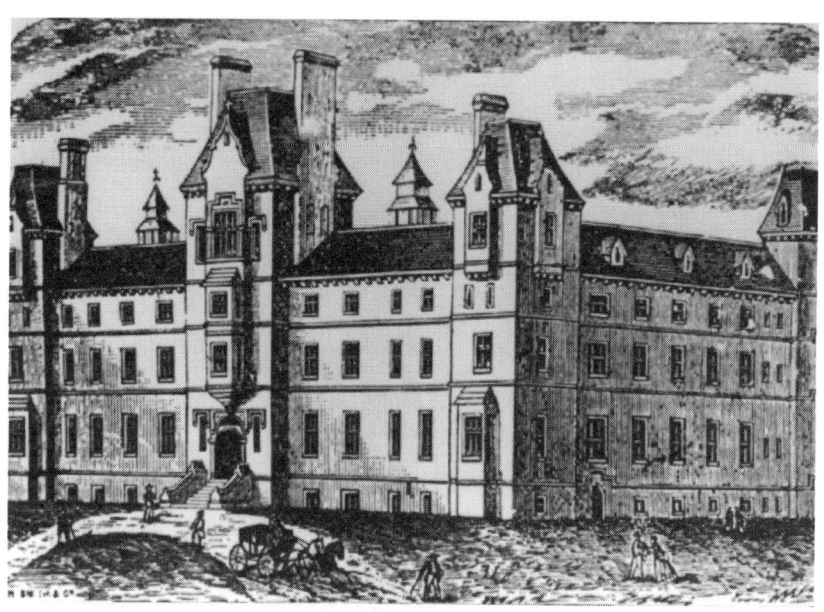

Toronto General Hospital, 1854-1878. (Spragge, from an old print.)

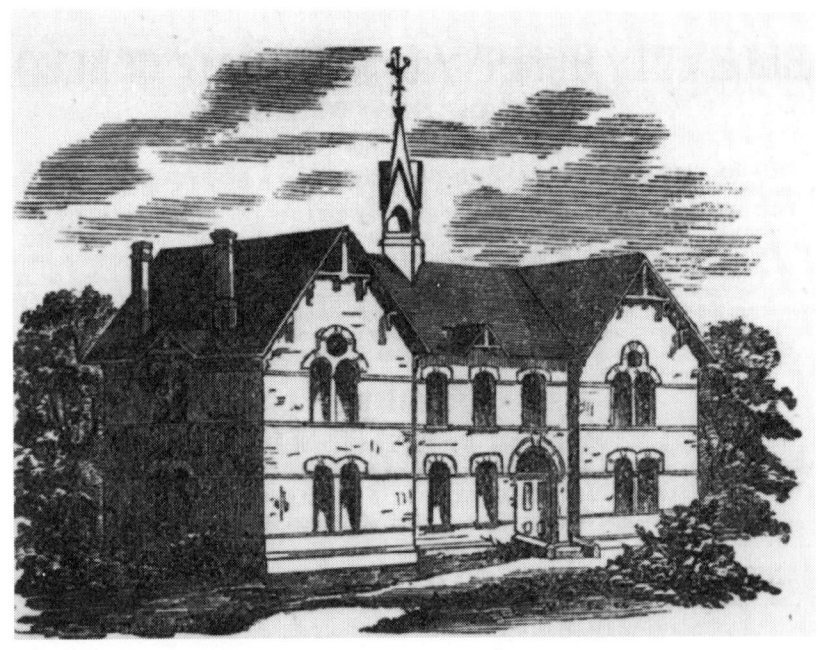
Trinity College Medical School, 1871. (Canada Lancet, Sept 1871.)

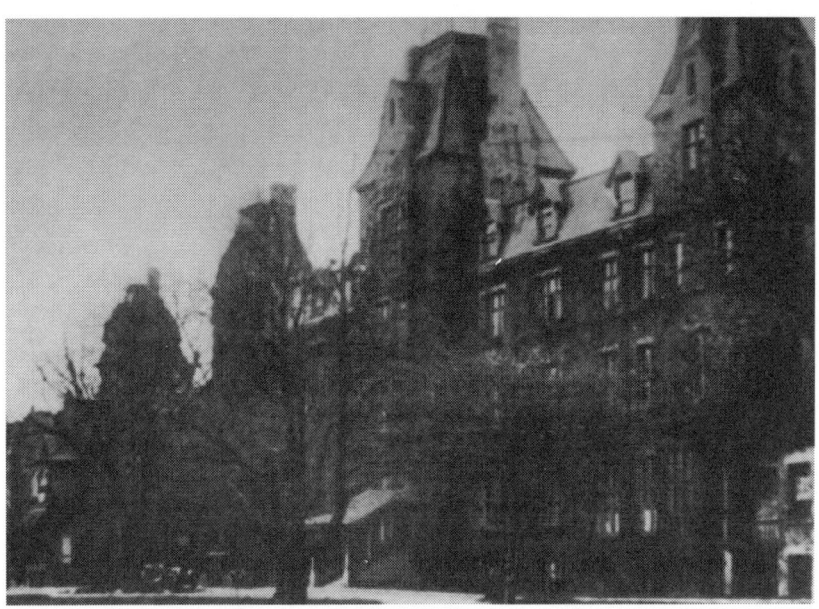

Toronto General Hospital, Gerrard Street, 1855-1913, (Spragge.)

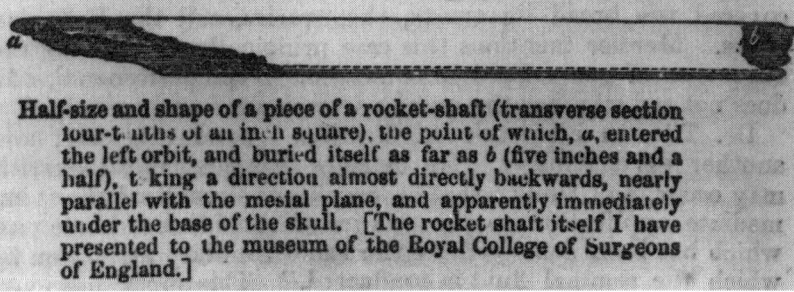

Rocket Shaft, 1862. (Beaumont, Lancet, June 14, 1862.)

well connected knowledge, and even more admirable in their order, their perfect clearness of language, and the quietly attractive manner in which they were delivered. As I remember them now, I feel that I did not esteem them half enough at the time. It was a great pleasure to hear them, and a good lesson. They were given on three days in the week at seven in the evening, after dinner. He used to come to the Hospital in the omnibus and, after a few minutes in the Museum, would, as the clock struck, enter the theatre, then always full. He came with a strange vague outlook as if with uncertain sight; the expression of his eyes was always inferior to that of his other features. These were impressive, beautiful and grand — significant of vast mental power, well trained and well sustained. He came in quietly and, after sitting for half a minute as if gathering his thoughts, began in a clear rather high note, speaking quite deliberately in faultless words as if telling judiciously that which he was just now thinking. There was no hurry, no delay, no repetition, no revision: every word had been learned by heart, and yet there was not the least sign that one word was being remembered. It was the best method of scientific speaking that I have ever heard; and there was no one at that time in England, if I may not say in Europe, who had more completely studied the whole principles and practice of surgery."[26] Doubtless Beaumont agreed, as he too practised the same care in crafting his later lectures in King's College in the 1840s; unlike Lawrence, however, he probably did not bother to learn every word by heart.

Though Lawrence probably helped Beaumont substantially, it is clear that their relationship was not just one of master and student. Lawrence admired the younger doctor's surgical abilities and was impressed with his inventive talents. He made liberal use of some of the instruments Beaumont invented over the subsequent decades.

After completing his studies in London, Beaumont embarked on a medical tour of continental Europe in 1826, a practice quite common with English medical students of the time. He began with a 10-month stint in Paris under the French anatomist and inventor Jean Zulema Amussat (1796-1856). Originally an army physician, Amussat became assistant surgeon at Salpêtrière Hospital, and later was elected to the Paris Academy of Medicine. In 1829 he published a prize-winning book, *The Torsion of Arteries*. Amussat was a pioneer in the rapidly expanding field of surgical instrumentation; in 1835 he successfully developed a technique for implanting an artificial anus. Four years later he was credited with performing the first lumbar colostomy for the relief of intestinal obstruction. This involved an operation to bring the end of the colon through the muscle and skin of the lower back.[27]

Amussat's skills as a surgeon, instrument maker and lecturer were eagerly sought after by visiting savants. Cooper, who toured Europe in 1834, visited Amussat and wrote in his diary that "he is a man of merit, industrious, and anxious for the truth." Beaumont had a similar reaction to Amussat upon his meeting with the instrument maker; their subsequent collaboration was very important to Beaumont's future as an instrument designer. Amussat taught Beaumont not only anatomy, but also mechanical and craft skills. He encouraged him to visit the local scientific and medical instrument shops, where his inventions were always prominently displayed. Amussat was impressed with Beaumont, saying that he possessed "un zèle et une aptitude rare."

Beaumont next went to the University of Brussels for a short period of surgical study before his return to England. Soon after his arrival, on 22 December 1826, he successfully passed his examinations and was admitted as a Member of the Royal College of Surgeons.[28] He was no longer just a student of surgery; he could now take his rightful place in the London medical establishment.

Chapter 2

Surgeon and Inventor

The fact that Beaumont had finished his continental education and had joined the Royal College of Surgeons did not stop him from continuing to learn. The London of 1826 was full of medical teachers and researchers, many in new fields of surgery, and Beaumont was far too astute to ignore such a golden opportunity. He decided to study informally under the physiologist Marshall Hall (1790-1857), who had just moved to London.

Hall, native of Nottinghamshire, received his medical education at the University of Edinburgh between 1809-1812. After two years as a medical student at the Edinburgh Royal Infirmary, he undertook his own European tour. On his return, he built up a large private practice in Nottingham over ten years until he moved to London, where he met Beaumont. The two apparently got along well enough together for Hall to start an informal "class" for Beaumont. Specializing in nervous diseases, Hall carried out his private practice and experimental researches from his home until his retirement in 1853. He became famous for his experiments into the physiology of reflex action, rational treatments of epilepsy, and his efforts to resuscitate drowned and asphyxiated patients.[29]

It is revealing of Beaumont's patience that he was able to study so effectively under Hall. Most doctors of the period found him "insufferably conceited and overly aware of his brilliance and capacity for work." One source admitted that "Hall was the most pompous little man I ever met." Pompous or not, Beaumont, like Thomas Wakley, the medical reformer and editor of *The Lancet*, was willing to learn from Hall and was one of his few firm friends.

Meanwhile, Beaumont began work as a surgeon in the Farringdon Dispensary which, being fairly near to St. Bartholomew's, left him sufficient time to visit the hospital and carry out his own medical experiments on animals. This led to his first publication, a 31-page pamphlet on bone fractures, which appeared in September 1831 and was received by a generally sceptical audience. This otherwise obscure booklet, however, is of great importance, for it gives the first hints of Beaumont's later promise as an inventor of surgical instruments.

The booklet, which was little more than a short pamphlet, compared different methods of immobilizing fractures in rabbits. He broke a rabbit's tibia and then compounded it so that the broken bones pierced the skin. He then applied a rigid dressing to keep the broken fragments from moving and to prevent contact with the air. After 25 days the dressing was removed, when the wound was found to be almost healed. In another experiment, a rabbit's right foreleg was fractured and nitric acid was poured into the wound. It was also sealed rigidly for 25 days, but by then an abscess had formed and had broken through the skin to expose the still broken bones; Beaumont sealed the wound in plaster for another eight weeks, after which time it had properly healed. He restricted all his experiments to animals, but he did advise extending them to man.

"I have not the least doubt," he argued, "that compound fractures, at least of the leg and forearm, may, in general, be made to get well."[30]

In his pamphlet, Beaumont describes an interesting instrument he devised to set broken bones. He believed that prolonged contact with the atmosphere retards wound repair and aids inflammation, and suggested instead that sealed casts of plaster of Paris would heal more effectively.[31] To accomplish this, Beaumont invented a specialized piece of apparatus to properly extend a fractured forearm or leg and hold it rigid while the plaster hardened around it.[32] He described the instrument as "a board, about 30 inches [76 centimetres] long and 18 [46 centimetres] broad, which I have made...[it] has a staple fixed at one end, and at the other, a strong piece of iron projecting longitudinally about nine inches [23 centimetres], to which is attached an apparatus of pulleys similar to that used to reduce dislocations; two pulleys, however, need only be employed, instead of four. In that part of the board, along which it is intended the limb should lie, there are cut several transverse grooves, about three-quarters of an inch [two centimetres] deep, and nearly two [five centimetres] broad; they are not more than an inch [2.5 centimetres] apart, and from three to four inches [eight to ten centimetres] long. By these grooves, the plaster of Paris, when poured along the limb, can pass beneath it, and connect below as well as above, the incrustation on one side with that of the other."

Had Beaumont confined his interests and inventions to animals, he probably would have had no enemies. But by suggesting that people could be helped in the same manner as animals, and by designing an instrument to be used in this way, he unleashed a storm of criticism. How disappointed he must have been when he saw the journals! The *Medico-Chirurgical Review* of 1 January, 1832, commenting on Beaumont's pamphlet, grudgingly admitted that "the common experience of surgeons has decided that a compound fracture is infinitely more dangerous than a simple one, and much of the mischief must undoubtedly be owing to the admission or contact of the atmosphere." Yet that was no reason to conclude that Beaumont's was right! "We do not consider it proved, notwithstanding, that this accounts for the whole difference in amount of danger between the species of fracture alluded to. Much must be attributed to the proneness of wounded skin and cellular membrane to inflammation." The journal reminded its readers that using a few animals was no assurance of success in humans, and concluded that of all the plans they had seen, "we do not think that Mr. Beaumont's will ever be generally acted on."

The October 1831 edition of the *London Medical and Physical Journal* was somewhat warmer to Beaumont, but it too had many reservations. It said the technique would only be useful on restless, irritable children, or possibly insane adults. However, it did point out that while Beaumont's methods had never been tried in England, they had already been successfully employed in Arabia, thus giving him indirect support that he would enlist a few years later.

The *London Medical and Surgical Journal* of October 1831 treated him no more kindly. While giving Beaumont credit for the originality of his ideas, it then went on to dismiss them as absurd and impractical. In its opinion, Beaumont "has as yet tried it only on brutes, and we advise him to halt there."[33]

Other journals were similarly critical. It seemed that Beaumont's first instrument was destined for the trash bin. Under Beaumont's prompting, however, a copy of the device was quickly deposited in the museum of the Royal College of Surgeons, where it was carefully catalogued and filed. But apart from this show of local support, it was largely dismissed by doctors as a useless and impractical toy. Yet both the instrument and the technique behind it did not die. By 1834 they had been revived by Berlin surgeon Johann Friedrich Dieffenbach (1792- 1847), and shortly afterwards, three English doctors also mentioned the device in a paper appearing in the 30 December 1837, *London Medical Gazette*.

One would have thought that Beaumont would have been pleased to see his methods finally gaining acceptance. Unhappily, this was not the case. People were now taking interest in his work, but they were not giving him any credit for its originality. Thus Beaumont was quick to respond to what he saw as an unjustified attempt to steal his ideas with a passionate plea for priority in the 6 January 1838 *London Medical Gazette*. In it he argued that "I may fairly claim to be the author of the plan," pointing to his instrument in the museum as evidence. Furthermore, he remarked that while many 1831 journals had unfavourably reviewed his book, at least none of them had questioned his originality. The *Medico-Chirurgical Review*, for example, had criticized him "without any remark that it had ever before been employed or proposed by any other surgeon." He also sent a copy of his 31 page pamphlet to the editor of the *London Medical Gazette*, and concluded his letter by challenging the editors to give their "opinion as to the plan of treating fractured limbs therein proposed; and also as to whether I am, or am not, entitled to lay claim to the authorship of this mode of treatment." Beaumont was evidently quite confident that they would see things his way.

Fortunately for him, he was right. The editors examined his work and admitted his priority. As they put it, "We have looked over the pamphlet above alluded to. It appears to us fully to bear out the observations of Mr. Beaumont." In the future he would not always be so lucky in getting credit for his discoveries.

Throughout the 1830s, Beaumont juggled his various medical duties with an ever- increasing schedule of experiments and instrument design. He had by now added to his list of tasks surgery at the distant Islington Dispensary, located on the north side of London, a duty he retained until 1840. He lived at 2 Manchester Street in Manchester Square near his parents' home in Marylebone until 1835. Then he moved to 47 Berners Street, between St. Bartholomew's and Beaumont Street, where he stayed until his decision to emigrate to Canada.

He continued to work at St. Bartholomew's Hospital throughout the 1830s. In 1834 he met the new medical student James Paget (1814-1899), who, with the German physician Rudolf Virchow (1821-1902), largely founded the modern science of pathology. Beaumont and Paget quickly became close friends, sharing medical duties around the hospital.

Paget had been born and educated in Yarmouth, Norfolk, but had moved to London in October 1834 to continue his studies at St. Bartholomew's. There he quickly made a name for himself by discovering the organism that causes trichinosis — trichina spiralis — in a human subject. The trichina parasite is a small worm which is usually found in the muscle tissue of pigs. Infestation is acquired by the eating of badly cooked, contaminated pork. The embryos develop in the intestine and spread throughout the body, but survive only in muscles. The disease was widespread in nineteenth century Europe, but the cause of the symptoms was unknown until Paget's discovery. It was an impressive feat for a medical student.

Paget graduated in 1836 and became a demonstrator of morbid anatomy at St. Bartholomew's three years later. He was appointed assistant surgeon in 1847, but, as was the custom, had to wait 14 years before attaining the full title of surgeon. He was a very popular lecturer at the hospital, which was one reason his surgical practice was so successful. He was elected a fellow of the Royal Society in 1851, created a baronet in 1871, and in 1877 was appointed sergeant-surgeon to Queen Victoria (1819-1901).

Paget was soon impressed by Beaumont, having special praise for his mechanical abilities. "I believe that few of our profession have equalled him in inventive power," he later wrote. He added, "Few inventors of any class have proceeded more directly to that simplicity which is essential to excellence." It was just as well that Beaumont was mechanically gifted; he was by now becoming quite busy at the various London dispensaries and he saw many cases that taxed his ability to perform operations with the surgical instruments available to him.

Beaumont was often frustrated with his patients' reluctance to see a doctor until the last possible moment, when they were often already beyond help.

William Clarke, a 63-year-old "debilitated and rather imbecile sort of man," arrived at the Islington Dispensary at 11:00 a.m. on 5 June 1834, suffering from a "tumour on the left side of the upper part of the scrotum."[34] Beaumont examined Clarke's tumour at 3:00 p.m. and concluded that "its form and situation were sufficient to satisfy me as to its being hernia." He attempted to reduce it by pressing on it for about 15 minutes, but was unsuccessful. He then questioned Clarke further and found that he had been suffering from this "tumour" for about seven years without treatment. He had felt no pain until about two days earlier, when a sharp blow on the abdomen had caused the tumour to swell in size and become somewhat uncomfortable. "The hernia having existed for many years, the absence of all symptoms indicating constriction of intestine and the degree of firmness about the tumour induced me to think it probably an old omental hernia, and perhaps adherent," Beaumont wrote. "Under these circumstances, I directed the patient to go to bed, to take a small dose of castor oil with tincture of senna, and in case of vomiting or pain coming on, to send immediately to the Dispensary."

Clarke returned home, took his medicine and went to bed, quite sure he would recover. Perhaps he was too confident. Ignoring Beaumont's strict instructions to come back in the event of pain, he passed a sleepless night and died early the next morning. He had made no effort to return to the dispensary.

Beaumont quickly sent for the body. He "found a common inguinal intestinal hernia. A loop of about five inches [13 centimetres] of small intestine was in the hernial sac, at the mouth of which the internal abdominal ring made firm constriction on the intestine, the coats of which were much thickened." From this we can conclude the herniated intestine was strangulated, which was something Beaumont could have treated had he known what was happening. He concluded regretfully, "If I had operated when I saw the patient, his life would very likely have been saved," adding that it was impossible for him "to perceive that an operation was necessary."

What was to be learned from this sad outcome?

"A patient who has experienced the least uneasiness from an irreducible hernia ought to be watched by those about him, even in the total absence of pain or other symptoms indicating constriction of the protruded parts," he wrote in a letter to the *London Medical Gazette*. Patients should seek help sooner and doctors should not delay operating "for the release of the incarcerated parts immediately upon danger becoming apparent."

Beaumont vowed to find a job where he could get to his patients faster. Military surgery seemed the ideal choice. In the early nineteenth century, many of Britain's finest young doctors enrolled in the army. Abernethy had suggested the idea to Beaumont back in the 1820s, and had recommended him to the Director General of the Army Medical Service, Sir James McGregor. Unfortunately, bureaucratic red tape had prevented the plan from bearing fruit. Beaumont repeatedly tried to enlist but finally abandoned the idea by the late 1830s after years of frustration. In the meantime, however, other opportunities for travel and adventure opened to him.[35]

To this period belongs the development of Beaumont's most important surgical instruments, including the one which is usually claimed to enshrine "the principle of the modern sewing machine." In 1836, Beaumont invented an elegant gynaecological instrument for closing fistulae; this was followed in 1837 by three new devices, a vaginal speculum, an instrument for removing polyps and his celebrated device for stitching in the depths of wounds.[36] Two of these, the fistula and suturing instruments, have been used to claim Beaumont's priority in the invention of the sewing machine.

Beaumont's fistula instrument was described in the 3 December 1836 *London Medical Gazette*. He invented the instrument "for the purpose of sewing together the edges of vesico-vaginal and recto-vaginal fistulae". He successfully used it in two of three attempts to close vesico-vaginal fistulae. He also assisted another London surgeon in using it and was understandably quite proud of its popularity and success. "The formation of the suture was not attended with the least difficulty," he wrote, "and occupied but a few minutes" in one case.

The instrument resembled a pair of forceps with curved blades, one of the blades mounted at right angles to the other. Behind this broad flat blade was a spring and at its tip an aperture; on the other was a needle, which held the sewing thread. "In using this instrument," Beaumont writes, "the operator has only to seize in its points, in the same manner as he would with a pair of forceps, the border of the fistulous opening: the blades should then be closed, and the ligature will be carried through one lip of the aperture. The opposite border is then to be seized; and the blades to be closed and held so. The spring on the back of the broad blade is now to be pushed forwards, by which the ligature is caught and held at its point. The blades are then to be opened and gently withdrawn, leaving a double ligature passed through opposite pairs of the fistulous aperture, so that a common or quilled suture may afterwards be formed."

Although it sounds complex, the underlying principle of its operation is in fact rather simple and can most easily be followed by examining the picture of the instrument Beaumont sent in. This figure clearly shows some of the concepts that were later seen as important to the germination of the sewing machine, particularly the eye-pointed needle; and if so, the instrument's role in the prehistory of the sewing machine needs more attention. We will examine this idea in more detail later on.

The following year, Beaumont modified the device into a more complicated "instrument for passing sutures in the deep seated parts, as in the operation for cleft palate;" in this form it resembled a sort of old style tonsil guillotine. Royal College of Surgeons librarian Sir D'Arcy Power described it in 1930 as "a straight instrument carrying a needle, like the present sewing machine armed with thread; the thread was caught by a fine hook and held as the needle was drawn back. At right angles are two flat jaws closing like a bracket and pushing down a slide. These grasped the margins of the cleft palate, and the needle carried the loop of thread through them. The hook held the loop as the needle was withdrawn, and on shifting the grasp on the palate and again protruding the needle, a chain stitch was made by the second loop passing through the first." Power was not the first to make the analogy with the sewing machine; once again, however, this is a question we will consider later.

This deep-suturing instrument also became quite popular among London surgeons. In his later tribute to Beaumont, Paget remembered that it caused quite a stir when doctors began to use it: "Of one of his instruments...that for the making of deep sutures...more deserves to be said. I remember seeing it used where it was first invented in 1837. Mr. Beaumont brought it to St. Bartholomew's and Mr. Lawrence used it for a cleft palate, and it answered well, as it did in many other instances."

A copy of this suturing tool survives in the History of Medicine Museum of the Academy of Medicine in Toronto. A gift from one of Beaumont's later students, the steel and brass device is signed with the maker's name, H. Hermann; although its end has been broken off, one cannot help but be impressed by the harmony of its careful design and intricate workmanship. The wear and tear on the instrument suggests it was well used.

Beaumont also devised an unusual vaginal speculum in 1837. In the early nineteenth century, both tubular and bivalve vaginal specula were quite commonly used by English physicians; Beaumont, however, inspired by ancient Hippocratic specula using wooden wedges, designed a steel bladed model that resembled an umbrella.[37] It was composed of five blades, each three inches (7.5 centimetres) long, attached to a metal ring one inch (2.5 centimetres) in diameter, the whole instrument being inserted with a rotary motion into the vagina. Each blade had a screw which drew them together by a string; after entry the blades could diverge, allowing a third of the vagina at one time to be exposed to view.[38]

Beaumont apparently constructed this instrument to further help him in closing vaginal fistulae; given the specula available at the time, it is likely that dissatisfaction with his "fistulae instrument" for vaginal operations directly stimulated this innovation. As he remarked in the 27 April 1837, *London Medical Gazette*, "I have used this speculum, and neither its introduction nor its expansion in the vagina has caused the least uneasiness. When introduced, it is wholly within the vagina; there is no handle or external part to obstruct the sight, or impede the movements of the knife or other instruments." These features made it popular with British surgeons for several decades, and it was widely illustrated in medical textbooks throughout the rest of the century.

Beaumont's other 1837 instrument was designed to snare polyps of the uterus, nose and ear, as well as enlarged tonsils. It was considerably more practical than the rough devices then in use. Its advantages included "a greater facility in applying the ligature, in its exerting a greater power of constriction, and in its being capable of being removed as soon as the noose is tied, without any diminution in the degree of constriction."[39] Beaumont used his new tool in three cases of polyps in the external ear canal and one in the nostril. He reported to the Royal Medical and Chirurgical Society of London on 14 March 1837, that "in all, the relief remains complete as far as he is aware, and in the three former instances the hearing of the patients was to a great degree restored immediately after the operations."

These reports and the case accounts of his "vaginal fistula" instrument formed the basis of Beaumont's next published work: *An Account of Some New Instruments for tying Polypi of the Uterus, Nose and Ear, and Enlarged Tonsils, with Cases*,[40] which he released in 1838. This was the last booklet Beaumont was to publish independently, though he continued to contribute regularly to the medical journals. In October 1838 he wrote a paper entitled "Exostosis of Scapula," concerning a very unusual operation to remove a bone and cartilage growth from a 13- year-old patient named John Reid. In this case, Beaumont eschewed his own instruments in favour of a small bone forceps (rongeur) designed by the Scottish surgeon Robert Liston; the patient survived the operation and was free of pain a few weeks later.[41]

Despite his successful practice and his reputation as an inventor of surgical instruments, Beaumont was still somewhat dissatisfied. He had been elected Fellow of the Royal Medical and Chirurgical Society of London in 1836 and many other honours were coming his way. Yet he wanted more opportunities to practise new surgical techniques rather than to collect awards. And his dream of military surgery seemed forever blocked by administrative red tape. Beaumont lost Abernethy's much needed support when his friend died in 1831, but he continued to apply to McGregor for a coveted army post, hoping that his stubbornness would eventually pay off. It never did, and his unhappiness festered. But what could he do?

Robert Spear was a student of medicine from Cambridge University who, after graduation, had joined the Royal College of Physicians in London and opened up a practice. Like Beaumont, Spear was dissatisfied with his medical career and was looking for alternatives. He studied the enthusiastic reports of colonization in the New World. Why not emigrate to Canada, Spear thought, and practise medicine there? After a series of abortive rebellions in 1837, the 1841 Act of Union had finally united Upper and Lower Canada; in the new climate of peace and stability immigration to the colony was booming. Furthermore, there was no more than a handful of qualified doctors to serve the half-million inhabitants of Canada West. There seemed to be no limit to a young doctor's opportunities. Spear shared his thoughts with Beaumont, and the two formed a plan to move to Ontario. They left England in 1841 and Beaumont's career thus far in London came to an end.

What happened to his instruments when Beaumont went overseas? Some went with him to Canada, but many others stayed in England. A few are still on display at the Museum of the Royal College of Surgeons in London. Those he took to Ontario were sold upon his death in 1875. Until the 1930s it was widely believed that they had been lost or thrown away, and that none had survived. Charles K. Clarke, the Toronto General Hospital superintendent, claimed that a copy of the deep suturing tool could be found in a box of antique surgical instruments at the hospital. Was this the same instrument that is now in the Toronto Academy of Medicine Museum?

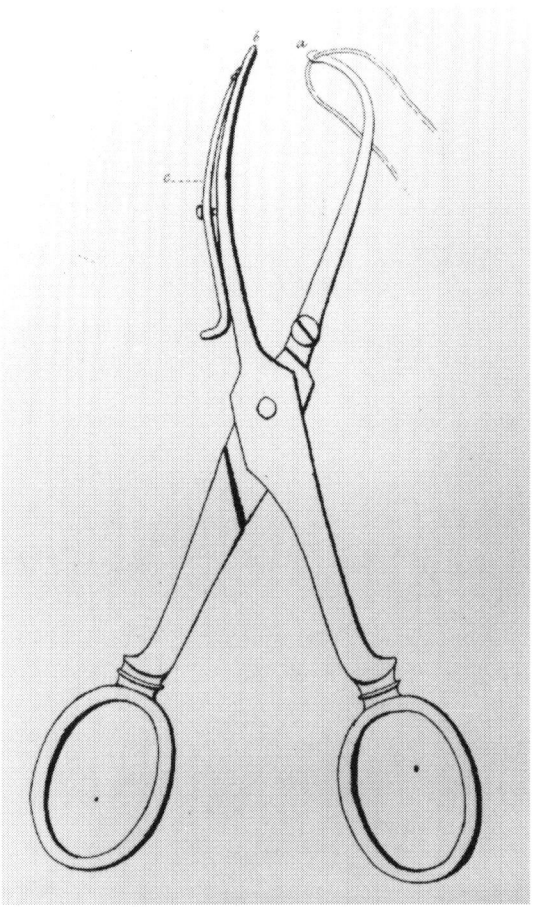

Fistula instrument, 1836. (Beaumont, Medico-Chirurgical Transactions, 21, 1838.)

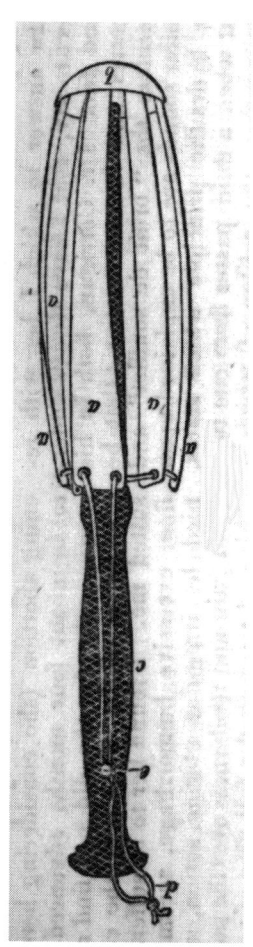

Speculum vaginae, 1836. (Beaumont, London Medical Gazette, April 27, 1837.)

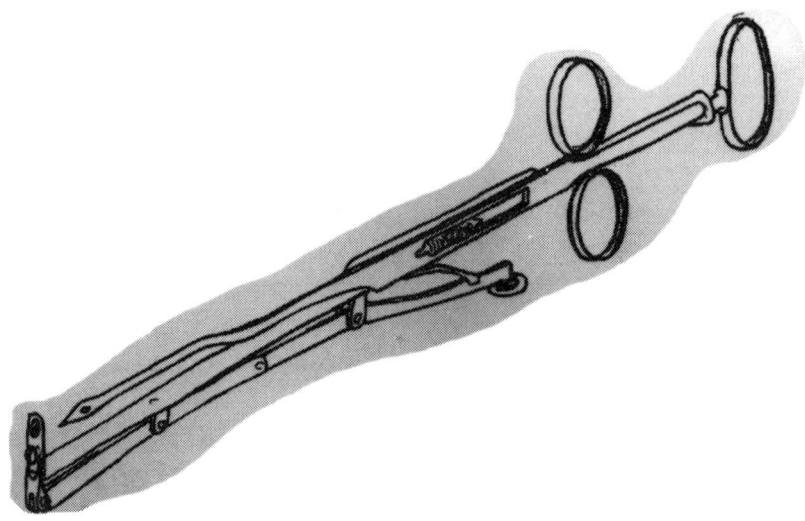

Deep suturing instrument, 1837. (Bell's Sketch, 1976. Original in the Toronto Museum of History of Medicine.)

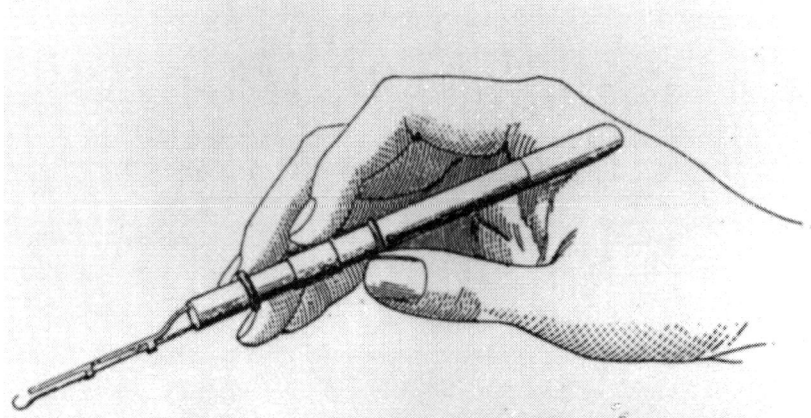

Manner of holding the forceps. The sliding spatula-like blade drawn back so as to expose the hook.

Iris forceps, 1863. (Beaumont, "New Iris Forceps," 176.)

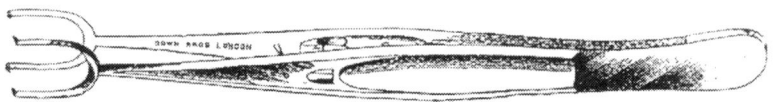

Fixation forceps. (Down Brothers., 1901.)

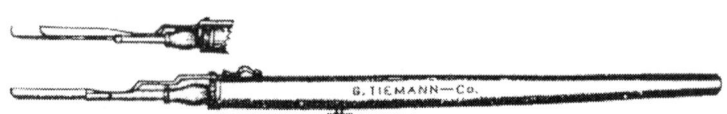

Canalicula knife. (Tiemann, 1889, 148.)

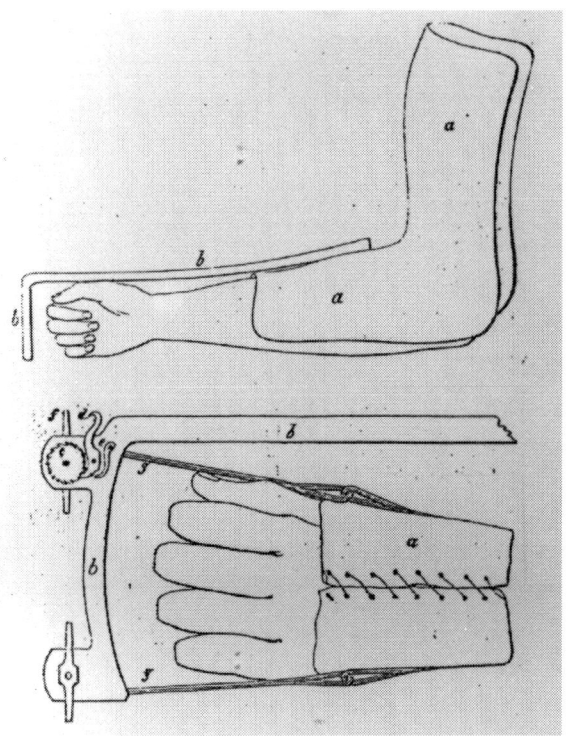

Fracture instrument, 1851. (Beaumont, Upper Canada Journal of Medical, Surgical and Physical Science, 2, 1852-53, 157-158.)

THE SEWING MACHINE.—It may not be generally known, but the fact deserves to be recorded in THE LANCET, that the principle of passing and arresting the thread in Singer's sewing machine was taken from an instrument invented by a distinguished member of our profession, Mr. W. Rawlings Beaumont, of Toronto, an honorary fellow of the Royal College of Surgeons of England, who used the ingenious instrument for passing sutures in vesico- and recto-vaginal fistula. Singer took his idea from Mr. Beaumont's instrument exhibited in the shop of Freeman, a surgical instrument maker in New York.

How the legend began. ("Medical News: The Sewing Machine, " Lancet, March 17, 1866.)

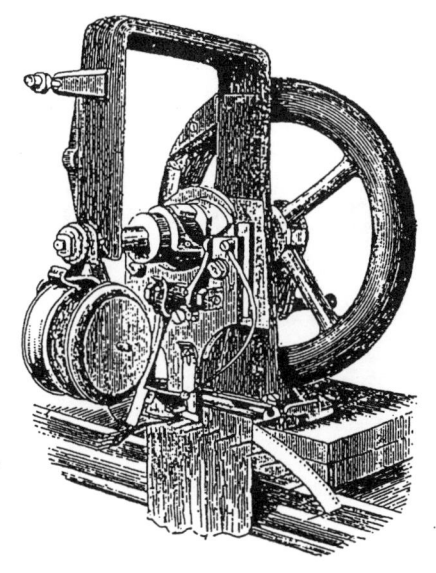

Elias Howe's Original Machine, 1846. (Chisholm, 744.)

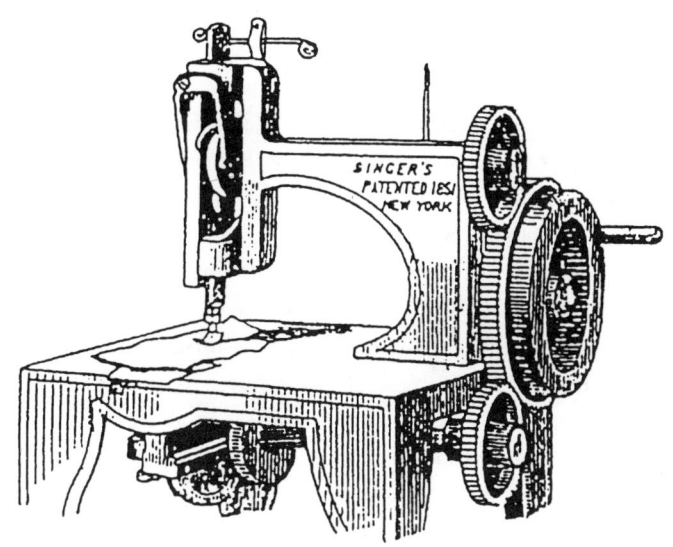

Isaac Singer's Original Machine, 1851. (Chisholm, 744.)

Chapter 3
The Toronto Medical Community

When the two physicians finally arrived in North America in 1841, they settled in Toronto (formerly York), Canada West.

What was Toronto like when Beaumont arrived? In his book *The Canadas in 1841*, Lieutenant-Colonel Sir Richard Bonnycastle (1791-1847) of the Royal Engineers described the city thus: "Toronto stretches nearly east and west along the shores of its spacious and beautiful bay, and consists of six parallel streets, of nearly two miles [about three kilometres] in length each, intersected by cross ones at right angles, at every two or three acres [about a hectare] distant, and the whole depth being less than a mile [1.6 kilometre]. King Street, the main artery of the city, promises to be very handsome; already many excellent brick stores and houses line its sides, and in the shops the superfluous luxuries of large plate glass and brass railings are beginning to appear. It is well paved with flag-walks, and a broad belt of round stone on each side, with a broken stone road in the centre. A capacious and very extensive sewer runs under the whole...The principal structures are the Parliament buildings and public offices; the English, Catholic and Scotch churches, the Methodist chapels, the Bank of

Upper Canada, the Market-House and City Hall, the Upper Canada College and Bank, and Osgoode or Lawyer's Halls."

By the time of Beaumont's arrival, Toronto also boasted a library, a new jail and courthouse, and a lyceum "with grounds attached, for zoologic and botanic purposes" was under construction. There was also a mechanics' institute, and a local literary club. As for educational facilities, there was a National School of Upper Canada, an infant school, a district school, and several common schools under the administration of a board of education. More importantly for Beaumont, however, there was the newly-established University of Upper Canada (King's College). It was located "about half a mile [800 metres] up an avenue in the centre of Lot Street," quite close to Beaumont's first Toronto home, which was also on Lot Street, and which he rented for £40 a year from Thomas Emmins. Indeed, as the university was the centre of higher education in the colony, he may have selected the house with just that thought in mind. Once he had settled in, he was ready to get out and meet his fellow doctors and their friends. Like all pioneering towns, Toronto's medical men were quite ready to welcome the new doctor from England.

At this early date in the city's evolution, the 20-odd physicians in the city of Toronto (serving a population of about 15 000) formed a very tightly-knit group. They served on the same committees, worked at the same institutions and, by and large, moved in the same social circles. As yet, there were few of the medical rivalries that were to cause so much bitterness for Toronto doctors a few years later. So when Beaumont began to work with the most prominent local physicians, it was inevitable he would soon meet the rest: Christopher Widmer (arrived in 1817), Henry Sullivan (1819), Alexander Burnside (ca. 1820), William Rees (1829), John King (1830), Joseph Orr (1831), William Gwynne (1832), Lucius O'Brien (1832), James McIlmurray (1834), Walter Telfer (1835), Joseph Workman (1836), William Durie (1836), Robert Hornby (ca. 1836), George Herrick (1838) and John Scott (ca. 1841).

Details of the lives of these colleagues of Beaumont will serve to paint a more complete picture of the Toronto medical establishment of the mid-nineteenth century.

Chief among Beaumont's colleagues was Christopher Widmer (1780-1858), one of the most important doctors in early nineteenth century York. Born in England, he was educated at Guy's Hospital and St. Thomas's Hospital in London, and entered the Royal College of Surgeons in 1803.

He then did what Beaumont had always wanted to do: in June 1804 he joined the British Army. The following year he was appointed assistant surgeon to the 14th Dragoons, serving with them in Spain between 1808 and 1814. After that, he came to Canada, dividing his time between Montreal, Niagara and York.

Retiring from the military in 1817, Widmer moved permanently from Niagara to York and was one of the members of the original 1819 Medical Board of Upper Canada. He gradually built up a large and well-paid general practice, and came to dominate local medical services. From 1822 onwards he was Medical Board Senior Member and President. In 1829 he set up a general hospital at York, where he was Senior Medical Officer until the 1850s. In 1839 he was appointed the commissioner to oversee the construction of a provincial lunatic asylum. He established a temporary asylum in 1841 and later on was chairman of the permanent asylum's board of directors.

Widmer was also the leader in local medical education. In 1834 he tried to establish a medical faculty at King's College, but Strachan's stinginess (he allowed only three part-time teachers) led to Widmer's resignation from the College Council in 1837. Sir Charles Bagot (1781- 1843), Governor of the combined colonial provinces of Upper and Lower Canada, reappointed him in 1842, whereupon he immediately tried to upgrade instruction at King's College. However, he quickly found that he was not able to fill the college rosters, and he eventually recommended doctors Gwynne, King and Beaumont, who had been recently trained in England. He seems to have been very friendly with Beaumont and was known for being very loyal to his friends. Indeed, it has been suggested that Widmer's high regard for Beaumont caused him to overlook the latter's professional failings.[42]

Widmer continued his dominance of the medical profession in Toronto throughout the 1840s and 1850s. He was chairman of the Toronto Hospital Board and its first consulting physician and surgeon. Considered to be very careful in diagnosis and treatment, he performed difficult operations at the hospital until well into his seventies, often assisting the much younger Beaumont. Added to his professional prominence, his wealth made him important in local society and resulted in his serving in several non-medical positions, including justice of the peace and director of the Bank of Upper Canada.

Widmer's private life was no less busy. Very popular with women, he was notorious for philandering and profanity of speech. He dressed smartly and loved to make hospital rounds in his riding gear. He was an accomplished horseman, and at the age of 61 rode from Toronto to Kingston without a break. In spite of his unconventionality, he was widely admired by the city's physicians. Indeed in 1853, as his life was nearing its end, even his bitter rival John Rolph (1793- 1870) wrote that Widmer was "still, you know, as he ever has been, and well named primus omnium." He continued private practice until about 1854 and died on 3 May 1858.

One of Widmer's first medical students was young Henry Sullivan (1805-1850), the brother of the second mayor of Toronto, Robert Baldwin Sullivan (1802-1853). The two were born in Ireland, but came to Canada with their parents in 1819. Both were avid actors who performed in several plays in Toronto during the 1820s, but eventually their paths diverged. Robert was called to the Upper Canada bar in 1828. After a distinguished legal and political career, he helped to bring about the union of Upper and Lower Canada in 1841.

Henry pursued medical studies. After an apprenticeship under Widmer, he returned to Dublin to continue his education, becoming an obstetrician at the Lying In Hospital. After moving to London, where he received a diploma from the Royal College of Surgeons, he returned to Upper Canada and was appointed surgeon to the Royal Foresters during the 1837 rebellion. He joined the College of Physicians and Surgeons of Upper Canada in May 1839 and was elected a Fellow the following year. Shortly thereafter he was appointed to the Medical Board. In 1843 he joined Beaumont at King's College as professor of practical anatomy. He also helped to run the King's College anatomical museum and worked in its dissecting rooms — and tried for several years to get additional pay for this extra labour. Unfortunately, money was tight and he was not successful until 1847, when he received a bonus of £50 from the college. He did not have much time to enjoy his extra money, however, before he died of consumption at the relatively young age of 45 on 6 February 1850.

Alexander Burnside (1779-1854) spent a long and active life in York until his death at 75. He came from New England uneducated and was considered by many to be a quack. He failed Widmer's first Medical Board examination, but tried again in April 1822 and was "found qualified to practise." He made a lot of money selling folk-remedies out of his Yonge Street practice. During the 1832 cholera epidemic he earned still more by providing clients accused in court of committing "nuisances" with "expert medical advice" defending their right to pollute the town! Still, in September 1839 he was forgiven and admitted to Widmer's College of Physicians and Surgeons of Upper Canada. He continued his practice throughout the 1840s, but gradually broadened his interests, becoming a director and trustee of a life insurance company. He died on 13 December 1854.

Burnside actually did more for Toronto's medical institutions by his charitable bequests than by his practice. His gifts assisted the creation of the University of Trinity College, where Beaumont was later to teach surgery. More importantly, his was the name behind the valuable Burnside Lying-In Department of the Toronto General Hospital, which his funds helped to establish in 1848.

The English physician William Rees (1801-1874) came to Canada in 1819 and first practised in Quebec. He moved to York in 1829, and the following January passed the Medical Board examination Widmer set for him and obtained his Upper Canada licence. He opened a medical dispensary in 1834. Two years later he tried unsuccessfully to create a provincial museum. He was also surgeon in 1837 to the 1st. Battalion, the West York Regiment. He was best known, however, for his efforts to establish the Provincial Lunatic Asylum. When the original building — a converted jail — was opened in 1841, Rees served as the first superintendent to its 17 patients. Eventually Beaumont himself was appointed one of its commissioners.

Rees insisted on the humane treatment of his inmates. Instead of keeping them restrained, he cut their chains and sent them down to the harbour for occupational therapy: fishing! Not all the patients, however, responded with gratitude to his methods and he was seriously injured by a blow on the head. The authorities seized upon this incident and removed him from his position. After many unsuccessful efforts to obtain compensation from the government, he died feeling bitter and cheated, in 1874.

John King (1806-1857) was born at Tuam in Galway and was educated at Trinity College, Dublin, and the University of Edinburgh. He came to York in 1830 and joined Widmer's Medical Board in January 1832, serving it until 1855. King was active politically, becoming a town magistrate in 1833. He was a vigorous proponent of public health measures, later becoming the chairman of the local Board of Health. In 1843 he joined Beaumont at King's College as Professor, The Theory and Practice of

Medicine, and taught there until 1853. He died on 12 January 1857.

Joseph Orlando Orr (1809-1869) was also born in Ireland. After attending medical school in London, Orr came to York in 1831 and served under Widmer as an assistant for several years. In 1840 he opened a pharmacy on Yonge Street, and in July 1841 he passed the Medical Board exam. He worked in Toronto with Beaumont until 1848, when he moved to Bond Head in Ontario, where he ran a flourishing rural practice until his death in 1869.

William Charles Gwynne (1806-1875) was another prominent Irish physician in York. Born at Castleknock, near Dublin, he was also educated at Trinity College, receiving his Bachelor of Medicine in 1831. The following year he sailed to Quebec as ship's surgeon, but by June had moved to York, where he quickly built up a substantial private practice. Throughout the 1830s, he opposed the ruling Tory clique that controlled medical licensing and education and by October 1838 had succeeded in earning a position on a reformed and expanded Medical Board of Upper Canada. In 1841 he was named to the managing commission of Rees' Provincial Lunatic Asylum. The following year Gwynne was on the examining committee that granted Beaumont his licence to practise in Toronto. Also in 1842, Bagot appointed him professor of anatomy and physiology at King's College, where he lectured with Beaumont from 1843.

Gwynne was on the King's College Council after September 1843, where with Widmer he led the minority opposition to High Church dominance of the college. Robert Baldwin's (1804-1858) University Bill of 1849 allowed him to stay on as professor of anatomy, but when the university's medical school was abolished in 1853, Gwynne moved to England. He returned two years later to devote the rest of his life to farming and the study of insects. Abandoning his private practice, he retained only his membership on the Medical Board. He died on 1 September 1875, during a trip to New Brunswick taken on account of his ailing health[43].

Lucius James O'Brien (1796-1870) came to York in 1832, the same year as Gwynne. Born in Woolwich, England, O'Brien entered the University of Edinburgh in 1812 and later settled in Kingston, Jamaica. Although his practice was very lucrative, he eventually grew tired of the hurricanes and earthquakes and moved to Canada to be with his brother, Colonel Edward George O'Brien (1798-1875). His timing was unfortunate, for he arrived at Quebec when the cholera epidemic was at its height. He established a practice on Yonge Street in Thornhill and joined the Medical Board in

1836. When the Rebellion broke out, he enlisted on the Loyalist side as surgeon to the York Volunteers and moved to Toronto. Soon after his arrival he was appointed Professor of Medical Jurisprudence at the university, and remained in that position from 1845-1853. He was also doctor to the local St. Patrick's Society and frequently saw Beaumont while serving as visiting physician to the Toronto Hospital. In 1858 he accepted the post of private secretary to Inspector-General William Cayley (1807-1890), and gave up his Toronto practice the following year to settle in Quebec. He died in Ottawa on 14 August 1870.

James McIlmurray (1800-1880) was born in County Tyrone, Ireland, and educated in England. He became a member of the Royal College of Surgeons in 1833 and came to York in 1834. He opened a practice at his home on Hospital Street, near Yonge Street, and became known for putting his patients' needs ahead of his own. On 14 February 1839, he joined Widmer, Rees, King, Gwynne, O'Brien and others at the Toronto Hospital in signing a schedule of fees to regulate doctors' bills. Fees in those days depended very much on just when and where a doctor was called upon. A city medical visit or opinion would cost five shillings by day, £1 by night. Distance also made a big difference; travel took a lot of time and doctors expected to be compensated for long journeys. For trips to the country, an extra tariff of five shillings per mile, as measured from the Toronto market-square, was added. Medical advice by mail cost a pound and five shillings.

By 1850, McIlmurray was also working as a medical attendant at the Provincial Lying-In Hospital and Vaccine Institute at 30 Richmond Street West. He continued his private practice, vigorously defending his right to be free from government regulation. In May 1851, for example, he joined Beaumont and other doctors in condemning a government bill that would have made all local doctors trained overseas pass a new licensing exam. McIlmurray was apparently very much in demand as a doctor and continued his busy Toronto practice until his death in 1880.

Another who protested the 1851 bill was Walter Telfer. Telfer was born and educated in Scotland, and settled in Niagara around 1826. He obtained his licence from the Upper Canada Medical Board in July 1833 and continued his Niagara practice until July 1835, when he moved to Toronto. He was appointed to the Medical Board, where he later worked with Beaumont. By 1844 he had acquired a large Toronto practice and was appointed as superintendent of the local insane asylum after Rees was dismissed. He held this post for three years, during which time Beaumont was appointed asylum commissioner. Like Rees, Telfer was himself removed from the director's chair after a controversial struggle with local government. However, he still had his practice, and by 1850 was, with Beaumont, an attending physician to the Toronto Hospital. He died in 1857.

Administrative stability at the asylum was finally achieved by the appointment of Joseph Workman (1805-1894) as superintendent. Workman came to Canada in 1829 and settled in Montreal, where he studied medicine during the 1832 cholera epidemic. He graduated from McGill College in 1835, but only worked a year before the death of his brother-in-law forced him to quit medicine and take up the family business of cutlery manufacturing. He moved to Toronto in 1836, continuing in the trade. He obtained his Upper Canada medical licence the following year, but it was not until 1846 that he got a chance to resume his practice of medicine. In that year he joined John Rolph's Toronto School of Medicine, which had been established in 1843 as a rival to Beaumont's school in King's College. Workman taught a course on Midwifery and Diseases of Women and Children. By 1849, he added another on Materia Medica. Workman was a popular lecturer and continued to work at Rolph's school until 1854, when he became superintendent of the asylum. He died on 15 April 1894, at the age of 89, having retired from practice 19 years earlier.[44]

William Durie (1779-1871) was born in Fife and began his medical studies at Edinburgh in 1793. Like Widmer and Rees, Durie shared Beaumont's dream of becoming a military surgeon — and was far more successful in realizing it. He joined the Royal Artillery as assistant surgeon in 1797 and became full surgeon in 1805. Durie retired from the army in 1836 and moved to Canada that year, settling near O'Brien on Yonge Street, Thornhill. He declined a position offered by Strachan at King's College and contented himself instead with a small consulting practice. Durie was a member of the Medical Board from 1838 onwards, but rarely attended the meetings. He did, however, appear at the important first meeting of the Fellows of the College of Physicians and Surgeons of Upper Canada, held on 13 May 1839. At the 7 July 1845, meeting of the Medical Board he was appointed with Beaumont to license candidates in "physic, surgery, and midwifery." He died on 14 June 1871.

The same Medical Board included the English doctor Robert Hornby

(1813-1869). Hornby was educated at the University of Edinburgh and was practising in Upper Canada by the time he was 20. In 1836 he began sitting on the Medical Board with Widmer and King, and for the next decade he attended its meetings. He was, of course, on the Board when Beaumont got his licence, and he consulted frequently with Beaumont when he joined it in 1845. Hornby also built up a considerable practice from his home on Lot Street, a few blocks away from Beaumont's house.

Hornby never seemed to be as much in demand as his rivals, for three reasons. In June 1839 he was accused of unprofessional conduct of an unspecified nature, but with the help of the Medical Board's other doctors he managed to have the charges dismissed. Secondly, like Rees, Hornby had medical disabilities of his own. "He was an estimable man and a clever physician," explained a contemporary observer, "but on account of deafness, he did not attain to the position nor acquire the amount of practice his abilities and acquirements entitled him to." Finally, he had an independent streak and sometimes fought with his fellow doctors on the Board. In April 1848, for example, he voted against Widmer, Gwynne, King, Beaumont and others who wanted all examining physicians to sign their names to the certificates granted to the candidates who took the Board's licensing exam. His opposition could not have made him popular with the rest of the medical community. Despite all these disadvantages, however, Hornby persevered in his Toronto practice until his death in 1869.

George Herrick (1789-1856) was another of the early professors at King's College. Like King, Orr, Gwynne, and McIlmurray, he too was Irish by birth. He studied at both Dublin and Edinburgh, and in 1838 came to Toronto, settling at 42 Lot Street, down the street from Beaumont's first Toronto address. The following year he became a member of King's College and got his licence to practice. In 1843 he joined Beaumont on the medical faculty, serving as Professor of Midwifery and the Diseases of Women and Children. His first lecture caused him much embarrassment, for although he had promised to speak to the general public about women's diseases, he was not prepared to see so many women in the audience! He soon recovered from the shock, becoming a popular lecturer among King's College students, who favourably rated his classes as "concise and thoroughly practical." In 1845 he also served with Beaumont on the Medical Board.

Herrick spent much time on the wards of the Toronto Hospital, where he displayed an eccentric bedside manner. He would act out the motions he wanted his patients to perform. For example, instead of the familiar command, "stick out your tongue," Herrick would put out his own, expecting the patient to do likewise. In spite of this unusual approach, he was well liked by his colleagues and patients and was on particularly close terms with King and Beaumont. When Beaumont, under the Hincks Act, was made one of the two university physicians to the hospital, Herrick was chosen as the other. He did not have much time to enjoy the privilege, though, for he died three years later, in 1856.

The last doctor in Beaumont's circle was another Irishman, John Scott (1816-1864). He was born at Strabane in County Tyrone, and like O'Brien, Durie, Hornby and Herrick, studied at the University of Edinburgh. He graduated in 1835 and came to Toronto around 1841. He built up a practice on Newgate Street until 1849, when he became superintendent of the lunatic asylum. He held the position no longer than Rees or Telfer. Finding work under the 12 asylum managers intolerable, he resigned in 1853 to resume his practice and, later, to become coroner of Toronto. He was another of the 29 doctors who signed with Beaumont the document demanding the government withdraw its plan to re-examine physicians already licensed in England. Scott died in May 1864.

These doctors were all an integral part of Beaumont's world. He worked with them, socialized with them and was influenced by them in varying ways. This is not to say that Beaumont ignored the important doctors who came to Toronto after him, like James Bovell and Edward Hodder, and others like John Rolph, who had for one reason or another moved away, only to return at a later date.

— Chapter 4 —

Lectures Composed with Great Care

One of the first things Beaumont did upon his arrival in Toronto was to apply for a licence to practise medicine in Upper Canada. He easily passed the requirements of the Medical Board of Upper Canada and Governor Bagot formally issued him his physician's licence on 12 November 1842.[45]

In 1842 Beaumont met the Cambridge scholar Dr. William Bulmer Nicol (1812-1886). Nicol had actually arrived before Beaumont and had passed the Upper Canada Medical Board examination in 1836 before settling in Bowmanville. Like Beaumont, Nicol dreamed of military surgery. During the 1837 Rebellion he got his wish and was appointed surgeon to the Northumberland Batallion. In 1842 he moved to Toronto and set up a successful practice. The following year he was appointed to the medical faculty at King's College, where he taught alongside Beaumont for seven years. Nicol was appointed Professor of Materia Medica, a post he held until King's College became the University of Toronto. He also became the Dean of the Medical Faculty and a member of Senate. In 1845 he joined Beaumont on the Medical Board and served on it for many years. He was one of the most active doctors in Toronto during the cholera epidemic of

1849 and received a special citation from the government for his efforts during the crisis.

Beaumont, meanwhile, built up his private practice. In 1843 he began to hear from Widmer, Gwynne and others about the possibility of a professorship at the newly created university. King's College had actually been founded in 1827, after Strachan had secured a Royal Charter and some much needed funds. The college was far too Anglican for the other religious denominations to stomach. Its charter stipulated, for instance, that the members of its governing body, and all the professors, had to subscribe to the Church of England's Thirty-Nine Articles. Upper Canada Methodists, Roman Catholics and Presbyterians would have none of this!

After several complaints about the restrictive language of the charter, an 1828 British Parliamentary Committee recommended that King's College be partially secularized. But it left supreme control to the Anglican Bishop of York, then Strachan, and stipulated that the university's president be in holy orders. This did not satisfy the critics, whose further protests led the Colonial Secretary, Sir George Murray (1772-1846), to suspend the charter. It looked as if King's College was finished.

King's College Council ignored Murray's actions, however, and continued to acquire land for the new university. By 1831 the situation had become intolerable and the Council was told to surrender its charter and lands. It refused, and spent the next few years fruitlessly looking for a compromise.

By 1836 it seemed that some progress had been made. The Upper Canada Legislative Assembly and Legislative Council agreed that the president of the college did not have to be a clergyman. Not only that, the Council members and the professors did not have to belong to the Anglican Church. A lot of progress had been made, but still not everyone was satisfied. The continued preferential endowment of the college with public lands was one of the long-standing grievances that led to the Rebellion of 1837. All the same, two years later Bagot finally authorized the construction of the King's College building and the start of classes.

As soon as the college was opened, local doctors began to plan a medical faculty. In May 1842, Bagot reappointed Widmer to the King's College Council to help select the medical professors for the new university. He was now faced with a difficult choice: should he try and make the college very prestigious by importing all the faculty from Britain, or should he hire some of the local doctors who were already available, but whose training might not be as good? At first he wanted to choose only professors from Britain, but eventually he admitted that "local interests must be yielded to," and recommended that the Council hire King, Gwynne and Beaumont. By late 1842, once the appointments had been made, Widmer left the Council. Then Strachan intervened, demanding a larger faculty. To prevent an increase in the salary budget, each professor would teach fewer subjects — and consequently be paid less. In addition to Beaumont, King, and Gwynne, the Council agreed to add Herrick, Nicol and Sullivan to the medical faculty. Beaumont was to be responsible for teaching the principles and practice of surgery.

He was happy at the prospect. After all, the money would be handy, particularly as he now had an extra mouth to feed. On 26 November 1842, his 21-old wife, Mary Catherine (1822-1866), had a daughter, whom they named Charlotte. The proud father had her baptized in St. James's Anglican Cathedral by the local clergyman and author, Rev. Henry Scadding (1813- 1901).[46]

So far, all this discussion of teaching work for Beaumont had been informal. Though it now had instructors available, the medical school at King's College had yet to be opened. On 25 September 1843, the King's College Council finally struck "a committee for establishing the medical school," which consisted of College Vice-President John McCaul (1807-1886), chemistry Professor Henry Holmes Croft (1820-1883), mathematics Professor Richard Potter and Dr. Gwynne, who had been appointed Professor of Anatomy and Physiology. They were told to "consult the members of the profession connected with the University, viz., Dr. King, Mr. Beaumont and Mr. Sullivan," to decide on the schedule of lectures, fees for students and so on.

By October 4 Gwynne had submitted his report on the medical school to the Council. The committee recommended that King's College medical students take "two courses of six months" in surgery with Beaumont. The fees for these classes would be £4 each. They would be taught in the east wing of the Parliament Buildings until a more permanent home for the medical school could be found.

On November 29, Beaumont was finally formally appointed the King's College Professor of Surgery and his salary was set at £200 per annum. The salary was comparable to all the other medical professors except Sullivan, who earned £250 a year for his lectures in practical anatomy. The extra £50 was for running the anatomy and pathology museum.[47]

Beaumont was clearly not poor. He spent a third of his salary on rent for his new house on 11 Bay Street, which cost him £5 a month. Firewood cost twelve shillings a cord, delivered to the door, but Beaumont required 30-40 cord to heat his non-insulated house through Toronto's cold winters. Fortunately wood was plentiful. Hay for his horse cost about two pounds, ten shillings for a tonne.

Food was inexpensive, but only if shopping was carefully planned. As winter approached, Torontonians would buy entire sides of beef and lamb at three or four pence a pound, which they would salt in tubs or freeze in the snow. In the summer, beef by the pound in the market was twice as expensive. Butter was a shilling a pound, potatoes a shilling a bushel, and bread was about eight pence a loaf. Because Beaumont belonged to a privileged group at the top of the economic pyramid, he could afford to eat better than most. Common labourers earned three to four shillings a day; skilled workers like carpenters and masons commanded six or seven shillings a day. Domestic servants received a few pounds a month, depending on their importance within the home. Beaumont, on the other hand, had not only his yearly £200 salary, but also income from his practice. A simple house visit was worth, on average, five shillings; for a more involved consultation, the fee was a pound.

The inaugural lectures of the King's College medical faculty were given on January 8-9 to a mixed audience of students and general public.

Thereafter, Beaumont delivered his hour-long talks at 3:00 p.m. twice a week in the Upper Canada Parliament Buildings on King Street between John Street and Peter Street. The medical students would hear Sullivan on practical anatomy at 10 a.m., then Gwynne on anatomy and physiology and Croft on chemistry. After hospital attendance and clinical lectures, King gave the theory and practice of medicine, followed by Beaumont. A student's day would end with various lectures at 4 p.m.[48]

Considering the number of students he had for his first class, Beaumont was well paid. In the 1843-44 session, there were only two students in the entire medical school, and only one — James Henry Richardson (1823-1909) — took Beaumont's course.

Richardson, a native of Presqu'île, began his medical studies in 1841 under John Rolph in Rochester, New York. He moved to Toronto and, after completing Beaumont's course, went to London and studied at Guy's Hospital for three years. After a short tour of European medical schools, he obtained his Royal College of Surgeons diploma, returning to Toronto in 1847. He began a practice and succeeded Sullivan as the anatomy professor at the university from 1849 to 1853. He also occupied the chair of anatomy at the Toronto School of Medicine, served on the staff of the Toronto General Hospital and was surgeon to the Toronto jail. He crowned his career by later becoming president of the Ontario Medical Association. Beaumont's first King's College student did his teacher proud.

Writing many years later about his medical experiences, Richardson remembered that "Prof. Beaumont's course of lectures composed with great care was delivered to myself alone. Of course we both wore our academic toggery, and the Prof. would kindly tell me to draw my chair near him in front of the fireplace during its delivery."

Richardson held a high opinion of his professor's surgical abilities. He considered Beaumont "in the prime of life, a Fellow of the Royal College of Surgeons, who had been selected and recommended by leading surgeons in London, as eminently fitted for the position. He was an accomplished anatomist, was perfectly versed in surgery, most pains-taking and correct in diagnosis, most skilful in the use of the knife, engrossed in his subject, and capable of communicating knowledge. He was the ideal of a surgeon."[49]

Richardson's praise was not confined to Beaumont's professional talents. He also had warm memories of his friendliness and personal qualities: "As a man he was most estimable, singularly polite, as gentle as a woman, neat in person, and possessed of the charity that thinketh no evil. He charmed all who came in contact with him."

It was fortunate for Beaumont that he was so well liked by his students, for all was not well between the medical faculty and the university's leaders. In addition to continuing complaints about the Anglican bias of the college, the administrators were also accused of meddling in the operations of the medical school. Meanwhile, the medical professors were having other problems of their own in the form of stiff competition for the few available students. On nearby Lot Street the rival Toronto School of Medicine was being organized by the controversial doctor and politician John Rolph (1793-1870).

Rolph always seemed to be getting into trouble. A native of Thornbury, Gloucestershire, he was born on 4 March 1793 and came to Canada in 1812. During the war of 1812-13, he was arrested as a spy but was soon released. He served in the London district as a military paymaster and then returned to England, practising both law and medicine. After a brief period at Cambridge, he went to London where, like Beaumont a few years later, he studied at St. Bartholomew's Hospital. He returned to Canada in 1821, was called to the bar and developed a country practice in Norfolk County.

In 1831 he came to Macaulay Town in York, where he taught medical students in his practice and was elected an alderman. In 1837 he joined the Mackenzie Rebellion, but was forced to flee to the United States when it collapsed. He stayed there six years, teaching such medical students as Workman until an act of Parliament granted the rebels amnesty. He then moved back to Canada and formed the Toronto School of Medicine, which was also known as "Rolph's School."

Alongside Rolph, Workman and George Hamilton Park (1826-1849) were a number of other professors. The popularity of their lectures soon began to draw students away from the more costly "live-in" medical program at King's College. This led to feuding between Rolph and Strachan, and Rolph's students soon found themselves having a hard time passing licensing exams. The reasons for their poor performance are not completely clear, but part of the problem may have been that most of the examiners, including Beaumont, were affiliated with the rival King's College.

Rolph and his competitors at the university, among them Beaumont, Gwynne and King, fought throughout the 1840s. At one point Rolph managed to humiliate the entire medical faculty at the university. Such behaviour, however, lost him many friends — and eventually cost him dearly.

In 1870 his school was annexed by Victoria University, whereupon the entire staff resigned and forced him into retirement. He died shortly afterwards, on 19 October 1870.[50]

Another, less controversial, doctor also arrived in Toronto during 1843: Edward Mulberry Hodder (1810-1878). Hodder was born at Sandgate in Kent and studied medicine in London, Paris and Edinburgh, becoming a Member of the Royal College of Surgeons in 1834, and a Fellow 20 years later. He moved to Upper Canada in 1838 and settled near Queenston for five years. He then opened a practice in Toronto, studying medicine on the side under Beaumont and others at King's College. He received his King's College degree in 1845, and five years later helped to establish the Upper Canada School of Medicine, which became the medical department of Trinity College, where Beaumont was later to work. Hodder received an M.D. from Trinity in 1853 and worked there for three years, subsequently joining Rolph's Toronto School of Medicine as Professor of Obstetrics. When he returned to Trinity in 1871, he was elected Dean, a post he held until his death on 20 February 1878.[51]

Hodder was a pioneer of obstetrics and gynaecology, subjects always close to Beaumont's heart. He helped to establish the *Upper Canada Journal of Medical, Surgical and Physical Science* in 1851, which later published some of Beaumont's articles. The two also worked together at the Toronto General Hospital and at the Burnside Lying-In Hospital. Hodder was one doctor Beaumont was glad to have as an ally in his later struggles.

Beaumont continued his work at King's College throughout 1844 and was rewarded on 26 August with his election as a Fellow of the Royal College of Surgeons in London. The honour no doubt pleased him, but the small size of his classes must have caused him some concern. Where were all the other medical students?

Some were simply not taking surgery that year. The college statutes required medical students to undergo five years of study, three of which could be at any recognized medical school, and only one of which had to be at King's College. For those who were at King's College for more than the bare minimum, Beaumont's "two courses of six months" could easily be put off. But that was only part of the answer: many other potential students were attending "Rolph's School" on nearby Lot Street.

Rolph's aggressiveness in running his rival school soon put King's College on the defensive. Not only was "Rolph's school" taking students from King's College, but the rival establishment was also making it difficult to obtain cadavers for all-important anatomy courses. Fortunately for Beaumont and his colleagues, the government eventually stepped in. Before 1843, there had been no formal way of obtaining bodies for dissection. Now, with two medical schools open, something had to be done. Act 7, Vic. C, 5, ruled that the bodies of people who died of exposure or who had been wards of the state could be given to teachers of anatomy (Gwynne) or surgery (Beaumont), barring any prior instructions to the contrary from the deceased.

This situation was better than nothing, but the shortage of cadavers led to a curious mixture of legitimate supply, purchase on the free and black markets and outright body snatching. Around 1850, for example, Dr. Thomas Deazley (1826-1854) of Grahamsville stole a body from the Toronto General Hospital and successfully concealed it in a barn after two policemen came to arrest him. Instead of condemning him, local doctors apparently respected his interest and ambition, appointing him to the Trinity Chair of Surgery in 1853. In 1851, meanwhile, Dr. King ordered an inquest into a questionable death at the lunatic asylum. It seems that a suspicious sexton had opened the dead man's coffin and found a corpse lacking a head, neck, right arm and right leg. The missing parts arrived three days later in another box, deformed by anatomical study. This case may have led to an 1863 edict banning the use of cadavers taken from the provincial lunatic asylum.[52]

By the mid-1850s, bodies, still in short supply, were being quietly "borrowed" from the hospital. In a letter to Rolph in 1854, the professor of surgery at the Toronto School of Medicine, William Thomas Aikins (1827-1897), remarked, "At the hospital Herrick, who is an attendant physician, gives over ALL his patients to Hodder and Bovell the two Trinity men attending...and until we get our Anatomical Inspector Beaumont and Telfer will ask no questions as to what becomes of their dead friendless patients, but it is quietly arranged that [they?] may go to Trinity."[53]

There was still some "body-snatching," though, as an 1855 letter from a Trinity College student shows: "Some of the students are medical, and as the bodies they require for dissection are sometimes stolen, we are all called 'Kidnappers'."

According to William Winslow Ogden (1837-1915), who later became Professor of Forensic Medicine at the University of Toronto, the practice of stealing bodies from graves continued into the 1860s, if for no other reason than the high price of cadavers. In 1860 they cost about £20 each, a month's salary for many medical professors — a small fortune for their students.

Beaumont may have turned a blind eye to the unorthodox procuring of cadavers, for he knew that a knowledge of human anatomy was one of the cornerstones of medical practice. He was critical of students who avoided his classes and hands-on dissections and he had little patience with examination candidates who he knew had taken short cuts.

— Chapter 5 —
Surgeon and Administrator

The Upper Canada Medical Board was established in 1819 to license the colony's physicians, but by the time Beaumont joined it, its mandate had expanded to include many other duties. Its quorum was set at three members and its original role was to "hear and examine all persons desirous to apply for a license, to practise physic, surgery and midwifery, or either of them, within this province, and being satisfied by such examination that any person is duly qualified...to certify the same...whereupon the Governor ...may, under his hand and seal at arms, grant to him a license."[54] The penalty for practising medicine without a licence was set at £100.

Thus in theory a great deal of power rested in the hands of the few doctors who sat on the Board. However, in those early years actual enforcement of the law was something else altogether. Many "doctors" successfully "practised" for years with neither a licence, nor retribution. Nevertheless, despite the difficulties inherent in enforcing the law, the Medical Board took a rigid position on medical licensing, and through the next few decades continued to demand evidence of not only high standards in training, but also in performance at the examinations.

The first meeting of the Board took place in York on 4 January 1819, with Widmer, Macaulay, Powell and the military surgeon William Lyons

(1780-1834) in attendance. The next day, the members passed the Hamilton surgeon and politician John Gilchrist and failed John S. Thomas of Markham.

In 1821 the Board began the medical examination of soldiers wounded in the war of 1812. Those ruled incapable of earning their living were granted "disability certificates" that entitled them to pensions from the government. For the next decade, the Board saw a steady stream of disabled veterans along with hopeful medical students.

Although many students made it through the Board's examinations, some did not, even after repeated efforts, and by 1832 the Board found it worthwhile to publish a list of requirements the province's doctors had to meet. First on the list was an adequate knowledge of Latin. A number of candidates had already failed the Board's tests because they were ignorant of the language. Next, prospective doctors needed to "understand Anatomy, Physiology, the practice of Physic, Chymistry, Materia Medica and Pharmacy, Medical Botany and Medical Jurisprudence."

Surgeons required a little less knowledge: "Relative and Surgical Anatomy, Physiology, the principles and practice of Surgery, Materia Medica and Pharmacy, and Medical Jurisprudence."

Midwives needed least of all: "the Anatomy of the Pelvis, its contents and their appendages, and Physiology, as far as it is connected with the same, a knowledge of the nature and treatment of diseases of parturient women, and of children, and of the necessary acquaintance with Materia Medica and Pharmacy."

These requirements stayed unchanged for over a decade.

In the 1830s the Board's powers were threatened by local efforts to incorporate the medical profession, but they were successfully kept at bay. Meanwhile, the Board continued to denounce untrained doctors practising without licences. After the 1834 cholera epidemic, it turned its attention to the promotion of public health. The Board also took an ever increasing role in the formation of a medical school at King's College. By 1840, under the domineering influence of president Widmer, the Board had a voice in virtually all aspects of medical practice, administration and education in the province. Other regular members at that time included King, Hornby, Gwynne, Herrick, Sullivan and Telfer.

By 7 May 1845, three years after obtaining his licence, Beaumont's success at King's College led to his appointment to the examiners' commission at the Medical Board. Now he would be able to question nervous

At that time, the Medical Board met four times a year in January, April, July and October, so it was not until 7 July 1845 that Beaumont actually sat on the Board for the first time alongside Telfer, Herrick, Nicol, Sullivan, Gwynne, Widmer, King and the recently arrived Joseph Hamilton (1798-1847). Hamilton was the only new face. Very little is known about him, but it is clear that he was born in Niagara and educated in Edinburgh. In 1835 he returned to Canada and set up practice at Queenston Heights. He came to Toronto around 1844-1845, but died in 1847 of typhus while attending its victims in the Toronto hospitals.

A proposal by Gwynne and Beaumont that not more than five members at a time be permitted to examine candidates was defeated, probably because most of the rest of the Board members distrusted the concentration of power that would occur as a result. (Although three constituted a quorum at the examinations, there was no upper limit to the number of attending examiners. Consequently some candidates had an easier time of it with just three of them, while others had to face all 11 examiners on the Board.)

Beaumont and his colleagues next turned to the more demanding business of examining the day's candidates. Six had shown up to be tested by this new Medical Board, which quickly showed that it was not afraid to use its powers. In contrast to previous meetings, all the applicants were rejected except G.L. Beard, a Pennsylvania-educated Woodstock doctor. Most of the candidates failed because of their "ignorance of the classics." One, however, was a member of the prestigious Royal College of Surgeons of Edinburgh, so knowledge of classics obviously was not the only criteria by which they were judged. Clearly Beaumont and the other commissioners were intent on elevating the level of medical practice in the province and had decided that a demonstrated uncompromising and rigorous stance at the outset was the best approach.

Candidates at the next meeting, in October 1845, must have been quite nervous. Were the examiners only trying to make a fearful first impression? Or would they relax now that they had flexed their licensing muscles? They did not have to wait long to find out. This time, Beaumont, Widmer, Hornby, Hamilton, Herrick, Nicol and King showed up — and failed all five applicants.

"The new broom continued to sweep clean," concluded William Canniff (1830-1910).[55]

The inability of candidates to meet stringent examinations on their knowledge of pharmacy, chemistry, anatomy, physiology, surgery, midwifery, paediatrics and many other areas was undoubtedly the main cause of their downfall. Frequently the difficulty was ignorance of Latin, which left the prospective physician unable to read several of the important medical reference works in the King's College library. Sometimes a political slant intruded: many of the failed candidates, for example, were from Rolph's school, whereas the Medical Board was dominated by King's College.

The bottom line, however, was that there were too many unqualified practitioners of a host of different folk remedies in the province posing as orthodox medics. The tough licensing requirements were intended to prevent "ignorant and illiterate men" from practising medicine throughout the far-flung regions of Upper Canada.

How much of this new Medical Board militancy was due to Beaumont? It was probably not due to long-standing members like Widmer, Gwynne, Hornby, Telfer, and Sullivan. They had been on the Board for years and previously had been more liberal in passing candidates. Other old-timers like Durie and King rarely attended Board meetings. The effective new members on the Board were Beaumont, Herrick, Nicol and Hamilton. The Board's rigidity did not substantially change after Hamilton died in 1847, and Nicol was reported by Canniff to be very kind to his students at examinations. So it is likely that the new standard in Medical Board examinations was due at least in part to Beaumont.

Beaumont's insistence on high standards from his students continued throughout the 1844-1845 school year. Coupled with his duties on the Medical Board were his lectures at King's College. He also had his private practice to consider. By now his name was becoming well known around Toronto and his colleagues were referring difficult cases to him. His advanced knowledge of eye surgery also meant he was very much in demand at the Toronto General Hospital.

* * * *

On 26 July 1844, Joshua Strother was admitted to the hospital for a cataract operation after previously having had his eye pierced with a needle by local doctors in an attempt to effect a cure, "by which operation no benefit had been derived," as Beaumont recorded.[56] He was immediately placed under Beaumont's specialized care. The patient was almost blind from a cataract in his left eye, and vision in his right eye was badly impaired.

On 25 October Beaumont operated on his patient. He used an instrument designed by the Austrian ophthalmologist George Joseph Beer (1763-1821), who was responsible for the flap method of cataract removal Beaumont favoured. As Beaumont described it, "I operated by extraction, making with Beer's knife a section of the cornea, forming a flap of its outer and interior half about one-twentieth of an inch [12 millimetres] from the sclerotica [the white shell of the eye]. The pupil being well dilated, I passed the point of the knife through it, and opened the capsule at the same time that I made the section of the cornea, on the completion of which, the lens very soft and broken in pieces, was expelled with a small quantity of vitreous matter." The operation appeared to have been successful and Beaumont put a cold water dressing over the closed eye and darkened the room. Three days later, he examined the eye and found it "very little inflamed, and the wound in the cornea apparently healed."

Unfortunately, Strother's recovery did not last. Around 1 November he left the hospital during the night and was found a few days later lying face down in mud. He "was brought back to the hospital quite imbecile, and having a cough, no doubt from exposure to wet and cold; still the eye appeared uninjured." Beaumont must have breathed a sigh of relief, but again things went wrong. By mid-November the eye was inflamed, and by 3 February 1845, Beaumont admitted that Strother's eye would likely not recover from the infection: "the bulging of the sclerotica had gradually increased, so as to form a good specimen of staphyloma sclerotica." There was nothing Beaumont could effectively do about this type of infection and "a paralytic seizure shortly after this terminated his life." It is probable that the infection had spread to the brain.

Joseph Wallace was admitted to the hospital on 2 February 1845, with a lenticular cataract in the left eye and poor vision in the right. There was also evidence of damage to the optic nerve. He had been blind in the left eye for two years, but had suffered no pain or inflammation. Beaumont concluded his 34-year-old patient was suffering from "a very chronic form of iritis, causing the contracted and adherent pupil."

Beaumont operated with Beer's knife as before. "With Maunoir's probe-pointing scissors, I then made two incisions through the iris, extending from the contracted pupil downwards, but diverging, by which extending from the contracted pupil downwards, but diverging, by which a triangular flap of iris was made, its base attached to the ciliary ligament. This flap of iris immediately contracted, so as to show behind it an opaque lens, which I thought could not be extracted through the opening thus made in the iris." Beaumont decided to try another incision. "I made with Maunoir's scissors a vertical section of the upper half of the iris, thus almost completely dividing the iris into nasal and temporal halves. Even now, moderate pressure failed to dislodge the lens, the uvea being so adherent to the capsule of the lens as to prevent its escape. With small forceps and Daviel's scoope, I broke up and extracted a part of the cataract, which was soft, and of a light greyish colour."[57] Beaumont again terminated the operation with water dressings, and gave the patient calomel and opium.

Six weeks later the rest of the broken cataract had not been absorbed, and the pupil had again contracted. He therefore "passed Scarpa's needle through the sclerotica, and with it further broke up the lens, and enlarged the opening in the iris."[58]

This time he was more successful and a month later Wallace left the hospital with vision partially restored, "the eye operated on being in appearance perfectly healthy." Had the eye not been so badly damaged, Beaumont concluded, he could have done much more, "as the operation removed all impediments to the passage of light to the retina."[59] Still, some vision had been regained and this case joined Strother's in a paper on cataracts Beaumont published in the *Upper Canada Journal of Medical, Surgical and Physical Science* six years later.

Difficult eye surgery like this and the many imperfections of the ophthalmological instruments then available inspired Beaumont to try to improve them. The results appeared early in 1845. On April 22, the Royal Medical and Chirurgical Society of London reviewed a paper from Beaumont on the formation of artificial pupils and his new design for an iris forceps. A summary appeared in the "Proceedings of Societies" column of the *London Medical Gazette*.[60] The basic problem Beaumont was trying to solve was technical. In the past, whenever eye surgeons had tried to remove a diseased or damaged iris with hook or forceps, the instrument would get tangled in the iris or the cornea, damaging one or the other. Beaumont modified the standard forceps so that when they were closed, the teeth were concealed and hence could not injure the eye. Beaumont explained that he came to understand the problem after examining a sometimes tears its way out of the iris, instead of detaching it."

With this modification, the instrument could successfully draw "any portion of the iris through a wound in the cornea," without causing further damage. With Beaumont's new device, "this laceration of the iris without its detachment never occurred, and he never failed, in any instance, in seizing the iris at the first attempt, and close to its ciliary margin."

Beaumont tried his new instrument on two patients. The first was a case of leucoma, "with contracted and adherent pupil, in which an artificial pupil was formed by detachment of the iris from the ciliary ligament." The patient's vision gradually improved to the point where he was able to work again. Before the operation, he had been able to tell only light from dark. The second case was even more successful. The patient was eventually able to read large print.

Although Beaumont's instrument was both simple and ingenious, Caesar Hawkins, who heard the paper, argued that these two patients alone were not enough to sell him on the merits of the device. Only one of them actually underwent surgery as difficult as the operations of Lawrence. As for the other, while it successfully restored the patient's sight, the instrument still ended up stuck inside the eye. "In only one of these cases did it succeed in completing the operation of separating the iris from the ciliary ligament," he reminded the Royal Medical and Chirurgical Society, "for in the second case the instrument somehow became entangled in the iris, and had to be cut out." Hawkin's point was justified, but in fairness to Beaumont it must be admitted that Hawkins was critical of many papers read before the Society.

Yet another patient, James Clifford, suffered from a capsular cataract in the left eye, complicated by a contracted, displaced and adherent pupil. In addition, his right eye was almost blind. Beaumont concluded that Clifford had a very chronic form of iritis.

Clifford's chances were not good, but on June 10 Beaumont operated. He began as before, "by making, with Beer's knife, a section of the cornea through its lower half circumference so as to form a flap of this part. At this point good luck came to his assistance. "The lens (almost of its normal transparency) was immediately forced through the contracted and adherent pupil, and through the incision in the cornea, by the mere action of the recti muscles, the laceration of the iris caused by the expulsion of the lens leaving as good and well-placed an artificial pupil as could have been formed by the most successful operation for that purpose."

Hardly pausing, Beaumont quickly took out the offending capsule: "the iris was easily ruptured, offering much less resistance to the extrusion of the lens than many an unadherent pupil. The opaque capsule, which was rather firmly adherent to the posterior surface of the iris, I extracted with forceps."

This time Beaumont's efforts were more successful. On June 14 he found "the sclerotic conjunctiva but little injected, the cornea slightly nebulous, and the incision in it apparently united." Five days later, Clifford could recognize a candle flame, and could distinguish the window from the wall in his room. He left the hospital with "vision somewhat improved, so he could distinguish large objects, and best in a moderate light." Six months later he could recognize objects in front of his eye and Beaumont happily concluded that the surgery was "as successful as the mere operation can be, i.e., the removal of the opacity without injury to any important part."

* * * *

Beaumont did not spend all of his hospital time working on these cataract cases. In 1845 he began work on "cheiloplasty," or plastic surgery of the lips. Two of his cases were published six years later in the *Upper Canada Journal of Medical, Surgical and Physical Science*.

The first involved 16-year-old Mary Ann Marshall, whose lip had been eaten away by a caustic substance used to remove a wart. An operation to repair the damage in November 1845 had failed. A second operation was also unsuccessful. On 10 January 1846, Mary Ann was placed in Beaumont's hands.

Beaumont decided to operate the same day. "Saliva dribbled from her mouth by day as well as by night; and the long continued loss of this secretion seemed to be the cause of the impaired digestion from which she suffered." It was difficult for her to eat and her distorted speech was hard to understand.

He began by cutting a semicircular flap of skin away from both sides of the mouth and dissecting away the scar tissue between them. The two flaps of skin were then rotated until they met. Beaumont then fastened them together "by two or three hare-lip pins. Union by adhesion took place between all the cut surfaces which were held together," he wrote. By

February 3, the new lip completely covered her gums, preventing the loss of saliva, and the patient was able to speak clearly again. The operation had been so successful that she did not bother to keep her follow-up appointments. She evidently "found her lips capable of all the purposes required of them," Beaumont sardonically concluded.

Hannah Shea, a 25-year-old patient at the nearby Lunatic Asylum where Beaumont was eventually to become a commissioner, had a mouth that was too small. She had been burned in the face and the scar tissue had reduced the oral opening to a small hole the size of a fingertip. A crude operation to re-open the mouth by cutting slits on both sides of the hole had failed.

Beaumont applied basic principles of surgery to avoid a repeated failure when he undertook the operation. He too enlarged the hole with a slit on each side, but he went a step further by connecting "the mucous membrane of the mouth (along the incision) with the skin of the cheek, by means of two points of interrupted suture, taking care to place one point of suture close to the posterior extremity of the incision. On the left side I did the same, except that I applied the sutures only in that part of the cheek below the incision, the structures above being so unyielding that I could not bring the mucous membrane and skin into contact."

Four days later the sutures were removed. Beaumont was pleased to see that the artificial mouth was working — though the operation was not a complete success. The left side of the mouth was tight from the earlier scarring and the lips on the left side had not healed at all. Despite this, Hannah's mouth was now big enough to admit a dessert spoon and she could talk without difficulty. Still, there was no getting away from the fact that the lopsided mouth was anything but attractive.

Beaumont decided to try again in November. He repeated the same operation, but this time cut out muscle and scar tissue so he could stitch the mucous membrane and cheek skin together, a tactic that was only partly successful. The skin and mucous membrane united successfully over the newly fashioned lower left lip, but not over the upper. Since at least one lip was covered — thereby preventing the mouth from closing up again — the patient was discharged "with the oral aperture of normal size, and shewing all her canine teeth."

Beaumont kept a close eye on her progress over the next few years and found the improvement was permanent.

* * * *

By 1846, Beaumont had become the one of the leading eye and mouth surgeons in Toronto. He had a substantial private practice, fulfilled his duties as consulting and attending physician at the Toronto General Hospital, taught students there as well and later on in the afternoon gave his surgical lectures at King's College. Fortunately for Beaumont, the Medical Department of the College was on the upper floor of the General Hospital, which at least cut down travelling time. On top of all this, Beaumont continued his active participation in medical administration, maintaining in the process his constant effort to remind the local profession of the importance of higher standards in the education of doctors. By the beginning of the new year his strictness began to pay off.

At the Medical Board's meeting in January 1846, Beaumont, Widmer, Telfer, King, Herrick, Nicol and Hamilton were in attendance. Before they examined the students, a surprising consolidation of power took place. A motion from King and Hamilton that Widmer should become president for life was passed by the Board. In their words: "Inasmuch as Widmer is senior in the Commission, and as such, by right, President of the Board, it is not necessary, in the opinion of the Board, that in future any election for President should take place."

It is not difficult to gauge Beaumont's response to the proposal concerning his close friend. On the Board since its creation in 1819, Widmer was now 64 and had always been willing to listen sympathetically to Beaumont's ideas. In addition, there was Beaumont's sense of obligation. Widmer had, after all, got him his first job at King's College. Beaumont almost certainly welcomed the idea warmly.

Beaumont and his colleagues examined two candidates for medical licences that day, passing one and failing the other. Success came to Thomas Clark Macklem (1817-1859) of Niagara, who had studied at the University of Edinburgh, and McGill College in Montreal. Their high opinion of Macklem was later confirmed when he was offered a job teaching in the Trinity Medical Faculty. He declined it because of his mother's poor health and instead spent most of his time at his busy Niagara area practice.

The next Medical Board meeting took place in April 1846. This time things got sticky for Beaumont and the other commissioners. There were seven candidates, four of whom were passed. Of the three rejected, one was "quite ignorant of the Latin language." This was Robert Hunter, a Whitby practitioner who had been trained at the University of New York.

Stung by his rejection, Hunter would strike back the next year. The successful students were Reginald Henwood, Michael Long, John Gunn and Henry Hanson.

Reginald Henwood's (1827-?) success was predictable. He had been one of Beaumont's students in 1845 and had also studied under commissioners King, Gwynne, Sullivan and Nicol. Moreover, he was the brother of Board Secretary Edwin Henwood (1819-1882)! He was later hired by the Toronto Board of Health to run the fever hospital for immigrants during the typhoid epidemic. He then moved to Brantford and built up a large practice, dabbling in politics in his spare time. Twice he was elected mayor of the city.

Michael George Long was also an obvious choice. He was from the small town of Aylmer on the Ottawa River and had been educated in Dublin. He had also taken the precaution of studying medicine at King's College. This gave him the same advantages as Henwood: the Commissioners were essentially testing someone who had already passed their examinations. Of course, it was just such a bias that so angered the professors at the nearby Rolph School. How could their students compete with this? But compete they did.

Henry Hanson (1823-1885) was originally from Cheltenham, England, and had come to Canada in 1844 and settled on a farm near Hyde Park, Ontario, in the London district. Later he went to Toronto and attended the Rolph School, passing with honours in 1846.

It is possible — and even likely — that the Board was more favourably disposed to King's College students, but a case like Hanson's did also show that the Board was not accepting or rejecting candidates solely on the basis of which school they had attended!

Hanson returned to his farm, where he built up a practice covering much of southwestern Ontario. There were at that time no qualified doctors closer than London, Sarnia and Goderich, so his territory was very large.

Robert John Gunn (1815-1900) was not involved with the Rolph School/King's College rivalry. He was born at Caithness, Scotland, and educated at the University of Edinburgh. Upon his arrival in Canada in 1842 he settled at Whitby on the shore of Lake Ontario, where he practised as a country doctor for the rest of his life. He was impressed with Beaumont's surgical abilities and referred difficult cases to him. Like Henwood, he devoted time to politics and eventually became town mayor.

The Medical Board meeting of April 1846 was marred by the problem of James Atkinson. The Kingston doctor had received his licence on 27 November 1844, having produced a diploma from the "Royal College of Medicine, London." This document certainly looked impressive, but it turned out there was no such college and the certificate was a fake. The Board Members sent a letter to Provincial Secretary Sir Dominic Daly (1798-1868), over whose signature the licence had been issued, warning him of the dangers inherent in licensing an individual who was, in essence, "detrimental to the public safety, and disgraceful to an honourable and learned profession."

The Board feared that its licensing privileges were being usurped. They had good reason to be afraid. Petitions had recently been sent to each of the colony's legislative houses asking for a reduction of the Board's monopoly over medical licensing. Herrick and Beaumont proposed that the best way to maintain control would be to ask the legislatures to send them any medical bill or petition for their expert advice before it was passed into law. Beaumont got the Board to send copies of this request to Senator John Hamilton, and Robert Baldwin, Member of the House of Assembly. The plea was successful and the Medical Board retained its monopoly.

Beaumont was by now becoming involved himself in local politics. A letter in the *British American Journal of Medical and Physical Sciences* a few years later claimed that Beaumont was one of the main figures in the scrapping of the 1845-46 College Bill and the Medico-Chirurgical Society effort to redraft it the following year. These two petitions attempted (among other things) to incorporate the medical profession. They were strenuously opposed by the Medical Board. Beaumont led the Board's opposition, which resulted in considerable criticism of his conduct.

"The petition sent to the Legislature in 1845-6, in opposition to the Bill brought forward by Mr. Sherwood (with the concurrence of the Medico-Chirurgical Society) was signed by Messrs. Beaumont, Gwynne and Sullivan, members of the Medical Faculty of the College; the movement originated with them, and the petition itself owed its paternity to Mr. Beaumont," a correspondent in the *British American Journal* charged. "The fact that Mr. Beaumont's petition has been the cause of the humiliating position in which the profession in this part of Canada finds itself placed at present, does not admit of a shadow of a doubt. To Mr. Beaumont and his associates chiefly the members of the profession are indebted for the insults heaped upon them by the tag-rag and bob-tail of the House of Assembly...but for that interference we should now have been a corporate body of several years' standing."[61]

Matters improved for Beaumont at the July 1846 meeting of the Medical Board. His colleagues this time were Widmer, Hamilton, Nicol, Herrick and Hornby. Out of the five candidates who applied for medical licences, four were passed. They were James Nichol, Gavin Russell, Benjamin Dickey and John Reid. Very little is known about these men. Nichol was a member of the Royal College of Surgeons in Edinburgh who set up practice in Perth, not far from Ottawa. Russell, Dickey and Reid practised medicine in Carleton, London and Toronto respectively.

At the October meeting, Beaumont and the others examined only one candidate, whom they rejected. So far that year they had seen a total of 15 candidates, of whom 10 had passed — a considerable change from the previous year, though not one that in any way indicated that the Board was loosening its high standards and rigid demands. Candidates were still being rejected for lack of Latin. Rather, the higher ratio of acceptances to rejections in 1846 was indicative of the improved instruction available at the two rival medical schools in Toronto. The students were simply better prepared and educated.

The same pattern continued into the new year. In April 1847, three of five applicants examined were found competent. They were James Salmon, Henry Lord and John Harvey.

English born James Moon Salmon settled in Simcoe, where he practised medicine and traded in real estate for the rest of his life. He studied under King and attended the Commissioners' classes at King's College, making him an obvious candidate to pass the Medical Board exam. Henry Lord, from Lacolle near Montreal, served as Provincial Cavalry Assistant-Surgeon. John Harvey was a country doctor from Kingston who had studied medicine with Beaumont at King's College.

At this particular meeting some effort was also made to standardize examinations between the various medical boards in Canada. The Toronto Medical Board wrote to its counterparts in Montreal and Quebec City asking for a "uniform system of examinations" and "the mutual exchange of the names of rejected candidates." After all, what good was it to turn an applicant down for a year if all he had to do was go to Montreal and try again the next month? Besides, the Toronto Board was anxious to enhance the profession's reputation by elevating the examination standards of all Boards to its own tough level.

The 1847 list of requirements for applicants makes very interesting reading. It includes, "1st, some acquaintance with the Latin language...if the candidate cannot construe some paragraphs of Gregory's Conspectus, a portion of the Pharmocopoeia Londinensis or a Latin written prescription ...the professional examination is not proceeded in. If the Latin examination is satisfactory then follow: 2nd, Materia Medica and Pharmaceutic Chemistry; 3rd, Anatomy and Physiology; 4th, The Theory and Practice of Medicine; 5th, Practical Surgery; 6th, Midwifery and the Diseases of Children."

A knowledge of Latin as a primary requirement for licensure was a carry-over from the British university tradition that the Board wished to perpetuate. There was a nostalgic belief that a knowledge of the classics was a necessary authentication of the educated gentleman, a label Beaumont and his colleagues were anxious to wear in the new land. But the Montreal Medical Board undermined these lofty aspirations of the Toronto Board and put an end to all thought of universal acceptance of the Latin requirement. "Our examinations are similar," stated S.E. Sewell, secretary of the Montreal Board, "with the exception of Latin, which C.R. Ogden, Esq., then Attorney-General, informed us we were not empowered to enforce an acquaintance with."[62]

The Latin issue came up again at the July meeting. Beaumont and the other commissioners rejected two candidates out of hand because they were ignorant of the language. They did, however, pass Samuel Seager of Walsingham, Alexander McDougall from Guelph, Charles Cameron and George Herod.

George Samuel Herod, who was born in Lancashire, England, was a Guelph doctor with a second practice in Georgetown, who had studied with Beaumont and the other Commissioners at King's College.

At the October meeting it seemed to be very much business as usual, but appearances were deceptive. Within a month, attacks from a former rejected student would rudely shake the Commissioners out of their complacency and lead to much public criticism about the way the Board treated its students.

Chapter 6
Scandals, Scholars and Sclerotica

Since its founding in 1819, the Medical Board of Upper Canada had enjoyed a monopoly on the licensing of doctors in the colony. There were many who did not make the grade, and as long as Board Members saw themselves as guardians of the public's safety, there was little likelihood of change. Why should there be? Doctors were happy, the people were content and students were satisfied with the arrangement...or were they? In 1847 one of the many candidates who had been rejected over the years finally protested.

On 12 November 1847, Robert Hunter wrote to the *Toronto Globe*, signing himself "A Newly Licensed Practitioner" and his letter was printed the next day. Hunter had appeared before the Board in April 1846 and had been failed because he had not known enough Latin. But that had not deterred him. On being rejected in Toronto, he took himself off to Montreal, where proficiency in Latin was not a required skill. He received his licence and returned home. Back in Toronto, gossip about his innovative accreditation filled the medical schools and eventually led to criticism in the local press. Hunter, embarrassed and upset, wrote the letter to give his side of the story.

The gist of Hunter's argument was that it was unfair to require candidates to pass a Latin test before being given their medical examinations. Had Hunter stopped there, he may well have scored points. But he went on to accuse the Medical Board of corruption and hypocrisy. Having failed his Latin test, he said that one of the members then offered to pass him anyway, if he was given a bribe. Shocked and outraged, Hunter rejected the suggestion: "And so I could have bought a licence from the 'Toronto Medical Board' if I had wished to pay £10 for it!" He concluded his letter with a scathing attack on the Medical Board and the men who ran it — and sat back to await their response.

He did not have to wait long. Three days after the letter appeared, the Board called a special meeting. They first wrote to *Globe* editor George Brown, demanding the name of the "newly licensed practitioner." Brown gave it to them the next day. On November 22 the Board wrote Hunter asking who requested the bribe, but Hunter stalled, replying on November 24 that "he had no desire to victimize an individual. I wrote defensively, not vindictively. Indulging a hope that the learned member who proved himself so devoid of honour and so unworthy of public trust, has ere this repented his gross abuse of the confidence reposed in him, and as giving up his name can only be productive of private injury and perhaps the ruin of an individual without accomplishing any material result, the writer prefers leaving him to the renovating process of time, hoping yet to see him rise from the wreck of moral principle."[63]

The Board was not sure what to do next. It forwarded all the correspondence to Provincial Secretary Daly at the end of November, hoping he would do whatever was necessary to obtain a "just vindication of the character and honour of this Board." The Board clearly expected Daly to side with them and issue a libel suit against Hunter. But they were sorely disappointed. Little did they know the provincial government! Assistant-Secretary Edmund Allen Meredith simply entered the evidential letters into the ponderous colonial bureaucracy and as they were passed back and forth the whole fuss appeared to gradually die down.

This was probably just as well for Beaumont. He was busy with his lecturing at King's College (he saw his teaching efforts rewarded in April when his students graduated; John Harvey, who had passed the Medical Board exam a few months earlier, was senior prizeman in Beaumont's course, and in the junior class J. Hagerman and George Samuel Herod both picked up awards[64]) and could ill afford additional administrative tasks.

* * * *

Meanwhile Beaumont's private practice continued to expand and, after a lull in 1846, his cataract surgery also picked up.

On 27 April 1847, Beaumont took John Duffy under his care at the Toronto General Hospital. The 52-year-old patient was blind in the left eye and had a capsular cataract in the right. Duffy could distinguish between dark and light but not much else and Beaumont sorrowfully told him "there was little prospect of improvement" in his sight. He was right: "I made a section of the lower half circumference of the cornea (of the right eye) and on endeavouring to extract the opaque capsule, I found it so firmly adherent that I could not detach it, even after piercing it and seizing it with fine hook forceps, and using such a degree of traction which drew the anterior part of the globe forwards. The capsule was so hard that when I pierced it with the knife it produced a crackling sound as if ossified. Some dark amber-coloured fluid escaped, and all attempts at extraction were ineffectual." Defeated, Beaumont placed a cold-water dressing on the eye and sent his patient home on May 22 "without any alteration as to vision in the eye operated on."

He had much better fortune three months later when a mysterious "Mr. A" became his patient. We know nothing about him except that he was referred to Beaumont by "Dr. Cobham of Trafalgar." This was almost certainly James Cobban (1802-1857), a Scottish doctor who had practised in Greenland and Jamaica before finally settling in Upper Canada in 1832. He set up shop in Trafalgar, between Hamilton and Toronto, eventually retiring to his farm near Milton.

Mr. A was suffering from a lenticular cataract in his left eye, but it was too complex for a country doctor like Cobban. Familiar with Beaumont's skill in this area, he sent his patient into Toronto to see him.

Beaumont operated on August 14 after having his patient rest for two weeks. The procedure was a complete success. In his words, he "made a section of the upper half circumference of the cornea, the pupil being moderately dilated with belladonna. Immediately the section was completed, the lens was forced by the recti muscles through the pupil, and into the wound in the cornea, from which I extracted it readily with the scoop."

He gave the patient a cold-water dressing and placed him in a darkened room for a few days. Beaumont was happy to discover that his patient could "distinguish even small objects." During an October 15 checkup, Beaumont found him capable of reading small newspaper print with a set of spectacles. Cobban must have been impressed indeed!

At the same time that Mr. A was being treated, Beaumont was struggling with a much more difficult case: Henry Fruin, a 36 year-old man who had been shot in the face in March 1847 and blinded in both eyes. He could barely distinguish light from dark in one eye. On August 15, Fruin finally limped into the hospital, where Beaumont diagnosed a blind left eye and a right lenticular cataract, an obliterated pupil, an altered globe and a diminished cornea. Fruin had virtually no chance of regaining his sight.[65]

Beaumont operated on August 24. As in so many earlier cases, he sectioned the lower half of the cornea and divided the opposite part of the iris. Then he used Maunoir's scissors to divide the iris vertically through its middle. Beaumont surveyed the damage and with a scoop removed portions of an opaque lens and a small piece of adherent iris. He then applied cold water. There was nothing to do now but wait.

Beaumont looked in on Fruin six days later.

"There had been up to this day scarcely any pain in the eye, to which iced water had been almost constantly applied," he wrote, "but to-day pain has been felt, and he was ordered to take night and morning 2 grains of calomel, with grain of opium."

This was a common pain remedy and it seemed to be effective in this case. Beaumont kept it up for a week, until the calomel made Fruin's gums too sore to continue. Unfortunately Fruin got no better. On October 6 Beaumont noted a "good sized artificial pupil," but admitted there was "no improvement in vision."[66]

There was nothing to do but send the patient home. Had Beaumont not had his simultaneous success with Mr. A. next door, he probably would have become rather depressed!

Beaumont continued working on cataract cases the following year with mixed results.

On 3 June 1848, he was given charge over John Buller, a 27-year-old man with a cataract in his right eye and a damaged left eye. Buller explained that three years earlier his left eye had been struck by a piece of red hot steel and was blinded. Shortly afterwards his right eye became infected and inflamed. By now, Beaumont's routine had become almost predictable: section the lower half of the cornea with Beer's knife; open the iris and divide it vertically with Maunoir's scissors; remove the cataract. He operated on June 8.

Four days later Buller was free of pain. Five weeks after that, Beaumont could see that a "good artificial pupil" had been formed. Unfortunately, much of the cataract was still trapped in the eye and Buller's vision had not improved. Beaumont sent him into the country for "a change of air" on August 22 and decided to try again on October 23.

"I found what appeared to be a piece of opaque capsule in the artificial pupil, and adherent to the cornea," he explained. "With Scarpa's needle I endeavoured to detach it from the cornea, but failed." He tried to push the opaque material back with his needle but only pushed the cornea back instead. Once again he had to give up and send the patient home. "He left the hospital without regaining the least vision," Beaumont lamented, "and I believe the eye became eventually disorganized."

Soon after he had failed with John Buller, 58-year-old John McNicholas showed up at the Toronto Hospital. McNicholas was a pedlar from Kingston who had begun to lose vision in his right eye in 1846. The left eye had been affected shortly afterwards. Buller was admitted on 29 June 1848 complaining of blindness in both eyes for four months. Beaumont diagnosed a capsulo-lenticular cataract in the left eye and a lenticular cataract in the right. After applying belladonna to the eyes to widen the pupils, Beaumont "made a section of the upper half of the right cornea through which I extracted with some difficulty the lens, which was large, rather hard, and of pale amber colour."

That was the easy part. "After puncturing the cornea and carrying the knife across the anterior chamber, the iris bulged like a bag over the edge of the knife," he wrote. "I withdrew the knife and left the operation on this eye for some time. Prolapsus [displacement] of the iris through the puncture in the cornea immediately followed, but the protruding portion was easily pushed back by the scoop, and the pupil contracting to a very small size, the iris was quite disengaged from the opening in the cornea."[67]

He gave McNicholas ice water, calomel and opium and let him rest. By July 8 he was feeling no pain and on the 27th he could see fingers held in front of his right eye; the left remained as blind as ever.

On September 7, Beaumont was pleased to report that McNicholas could "read ordinary print with a proper glass," though he was aware that his patient was by no means out of the woods. The right eye still showed some slight remains of cataract and the left remained stubbornly useless. On September 15, Beaumont made an incision in the left eye. This time "the cataract was expelled immediately on the completion of the incision, with some vitreous humour, but without any prolapsus of the iris, as in the first attempt." The patient recovered speedily and by October 1 he could see fingers held in front of either eye. Beaumont sent him home a few weeks later, "having tolerably good vision of both eyes, but best of that first operated on. A few things, he said, appeared to him double, as in the flame of a candle and the moon, but he could read ordinary print without any appearance of the letters or lines being indistinct or double."

Beaumont's progress in the treatment of difficult cataract cases had unexpected benefits. Frequently the town's most important citizens would seek him out for his advice on medical matters. No less a figure than Bishop Strachan counted himself among Beaumont's patients and sent him a £5 cheque for his services.[68]

Beaumont hardly needed the money, but the encouraging letter that Strachan had also included must have helped combat the depressing effects of the ongoing Hunter affair that continued to plague the Medical Board.

* * * *

Despite the dampening effects of the administrative paper-shuffle at government level, Toronto remained abuzz with talk of the scandal. It was bad enough that a Board Member was rumoured to have been willing to pass a failing candidate for £10, but what was even more incredible was that Hunter, a fellow practitioner, had actually publicly chastised the Board in the pages of the *Globe* — and, worse, gotten away with it. The Board seemed to be doing nothing to restore its good name.

Beaumont and the commissioners entered 1848 profoundly dissatisfied with the government's inaction on their behalf. It might have occurred to them to stop licensing doctors until the Colony acted, but that would have deprived them of their main bargaining tool, so the Board continued to fulfil its mandate.

In January 1848, Beaumont and the others passed two applicants: Godfrey Schmutter and Joshua Fidlar.

Godfrey H. Schmutter was a doctor from Berlin who showed the Board a Prussian Doctor of Medicine and Surgery diploma. Joshua Fidlar was a country doctor from Lindsay.[69]

In April, another 11 candidates came forward, but only six were successful. They included William H. Wilson (Simcoe), William Scott (Woodstock), David Farrar (London), John Phelan (Toronto) and Edward Hipkins of Richmond Hill. The last to present himself was George Holmes (Perth), who was a member of Dublin's Royal College of Surgeons and was also an assistant to the Plymouth Royal Marine Hospital.

By now, Beaumont was clearly getting fed up, and the April meeting finally saw efforts at damage control in the Hunter affair. Gwynne and Sullivan were asked to find out from Baldwin what the government intended to do about the "libellous attacks upon the Board." In addition, the Board decided to write the names of examining Commissioners on candidates' certificates. That way everyone would know who passed a given student. It wouldn't remove the accusation of corruption, but at least it would make Board members a little more accountable. Beaumont and five others voted in favour of the resolution.

The only opposing voice was Hornby's. Could he have been the one who asked Hunter for the bribe? After all, it was not the first time he had been accused of improper conduct. An earlier charge had been thrown out in 1839 with the help of the other Board members.

On July 3, the Board heard of more government stonewalling from Baldwin. He told them that the Attorney-General had looked at the Hunter papers and had written a report (which had subsequently been lost in the files of the bureaucracy!) advising against proceeding with an action for libel and instead to be patient since "the subject has not been forgotten."

Whether that was true or not, the fact remained that the Colony had little to gain and everything to lose by assuaging the Board's wounded pride. Furthermore, dragging the whole mess through the courts would accomplish little. At best, it would give the Board a hollow triumph, for the damage to its reputation had already been done. And what if it lost? What if more disgruntled medical students came forward? How would the Colony's prized Medical Board face them? No, it was probably better to let the whole affair drop.

To make matters worse, at the same July meeting Secretary Edwin Henwood, a friend of Beaumont's, announced that he was leaving the Board to move to Hamilton (where he later became surgeon to the local hospital). He was replaced by Toronto General Hospital house surgeon Edward Clarke.

There were seven medical licence applications in July, of which two failed. Beaumont and his colleagues gave certificates to Egerton Perry of Cobourg and Samuel Sedden Woolbank, Horace Croft Hastings, William Case Wright and John Clark Wasbrick, all of Toronto.

* * * *

1848 also saw an unrelated development in the medical community with the arrival in Toronto of the Church of England clergyman, scholar and physician James Bovell (1817-1880). Born in Barbados, Bovell studied medicine at Guy's Hospital. Like Beaumont, he became a dresser, this time for Astley Cooper. He also studied medicine at Glasgow and Edinburgh — finally graduating in 1839 — and then practised in Barbados before his move to Upper Canada.[70]

In Toronto he became one of the city's most important physicians, closely associated with Beaumont and Hodder, the three making use of each others' specialized skills. He joined Hodder at the newly-formed medical faculty of Trinity College and co-founded the *Upper Canada Journal of Medical, Surgical and Physical Science*, which would later print many of Beaumont's clinical case studies.

Bovell played an important part in treating victims of the cholera epidemic of 1854. He appreciated that the chief danger of cholera was dehydration and took steps to correct it, thereby saving many more lives than might otherwise have been expected.

Between 1857 and 1870 Bovell taught physiology, chemistry and natural theology at Trinity, where one of his students was William Osler. In 1870 he returned to the West Indies, where he died from a stroke in 1880.

Bovell had not been in Toronto long before he was drawn into local medical politics. The feuding between King's College and the Toronto School of Medicine was still very much alive, with no sign of compromise on either side. Bovell and Hodder stepped right into this fray by proposing yet another medical school, which came into being in 1850.

* * * *

In 1849 two new doctors were licensed who were to become famous and have an impact upon the practice of medicine in Ontario: William Thomas Aikins (1827-1897) and Uzziel Ogden (1827- 1909).

Beaumont was to regret his decision to pass the first of these candidates when Aikins became a bitter rival who attempted to unseat him at the Toronto Hospital a few years later. Aikins was educated at Jefferson Medical College in Philadelphia, but he also attended classes at the Rolph School, where he became anatomy instructor in 1850.

It was Aikins who took control of the school in 1856 with the other lecturers and established himself as president, a position he held until 1887 when he created the University of Toronto medical faculty from the remains of his Toronto School of Medicine. Aikins went on to served as dean of the faculty until 1893. He also served as a leading member of the Council of the Ontario College of Physicians and Surgeons. He died on 25 May 1897.[71]

Ogden was born in Toronto and was educated at the Toronto School of Medicine. He earned his M.D. degree from the University of Victoria College in 1855 and became the editor of one of the early medical journals in Upper Canada, the *Canadian Practitioner*.

Ogden built up a thriving practice in Toronto, much of it concerned with a field Beaumont had also long been interested in: obstetrics and the diseases of women. Unlike Aikins, however, he did not see himself as a rival to Beaumont and he eventually became gynaecology professor at the University of Toronto.

* * * *

By the end of 1849, Beaumont and his colleagues had examined 21 students and had passed 14. Things had improved at the Medical Board. The Hunter controversy had died down again, more applicants were passing and, importantly, candidates from the Toronto School of Medicine were having more success. This may have been a reaction to the charges of bias, but an equal share of the credit should go to Rolph himself, who worked relentlessly to improve instruction and facilities at his school.

Beaumont once again had his hands full with cataract patients at the Toronto Hospital, his native ingenuity serving him well when confronted with difficult technical decisions in the operating room. Thus, whenever the situation demanded it, he would either modify an existing device or invent a new one altogether.

He wrote in one operation that he had used "a fine and much curved Scarpa's needle, the cutting edges rounded off, to within one-tenth of an inch [a quarter of a centimetre] of its point."[72]

Sometimes his innovations were successful, at other times, not. This particular adaptation, for example, failed to help one Hugh King, though the instrument itself served well: "The cornea was easily pierced," he wrote, "and the lens and its capsule freely divided, as well as some of the adhesions of the iris." Having pushed the needle through the cornea, he twisted it "so as to bring its [the needle's] convex surface towards the cornea, and then entering the point deeply into the lens, I divided it and the capsule freely. On withdrawing the needle, I rotated it back again, so as to bring its convex surface again towards the iris."

Beaumont looked in on King six days later. The result was "of little value," he frankly concluded, "owing to the great impairment of the nervous apparatus of vision."

It did help, on the other hand, a patient who had cataracts in both eyes "from the great and long-continued inflammation succeeding to these operations" at the hands of other surgeons. John Bolding, 72, could barely distinguish light from dark when Beaumont decided to operate.

With his modified needle, he "separated the adhesions, which broke readily, and having lacerated the capsule, I divided the lens into several pieces, some of which escaped into the anterior chamber." For two weeks Bolding recovered and was free of inflammation, but then Beaumont discovered pus had collected in the lower part of the anterior chamber. Operating again, he "made a section of the lower third of the cornea, through which the deposit (semi-fluid) immediately escaped, and most of the remains of the cataract I removed with the scoop and toothed forceps." This was the instrument he had created a few years earlier. A month later there was "no pain, and very little inflammation." In a good light Bolding could now see the bars of his window.

Beaumont continued his cataract work at the Toronto Hospital into the following year.

Robert Simpson, a 21-year-old diabetic, was stricken with cataracts in both eyes. Fortunately his general vision was still relatively good and there was as yet little structural damage. After dilating the iris with belladonna, Beaumont incised the lower half of the cornea, simultaneously dividing the capsule of the lens. Everything almost went dreadfully wrong when Simpson panicked and in the ensuing pandemonium Beaumont lost control of his knife. As he explained later: "The patient seized my arm at the time the knife was passing across the anterior chamber, which caused its point to wound slightly the nasal and lower side of the pupillary margin of the iris. The cataract broken up, escaped at once, with some protrusion of the iris."

Beaumont pulled the eyelid over the protruding iris and gently massaged it, and all was well. A month after the operation, Simpson was reading with the aid of a convex glass. A successful operation on the right eye followed — accompanied by a reduction in the patient's meat ration to ensure a less stimulating diet.

* * * *

By the end of the 1840s Beaumont had become the leading eye surgeon of Toronto and had built up a large referral practice. His work brought him praise from his patients and, more importantly, warm recommendations from other colleagues, particularly Hodder and Bovell.

He attended to his duties at the Medical Board admirably, putting applicants through rigorous examinations and taking an active role at Board meetings.

Also, in addition to teaching at King's College, he had begun to participate in college politics and administration.

—— Chapter 7 ——
Medical Schools at War

By the late 1840s Beaumont was well established as an important and influential figure in the Toronto medical community. On 27 September 1848, he became a member of King's College Council and thus was able to expanded his sphere of influence to include university policy. He was quick to make use of the opportunity.

By the fall of 1848 Beaumont had become a regular and vocal attendee at King's College Council meetings, sometimes to the dismay of university leaders. On September 30, Beaumont and Gwynne proposed that the College stop subsidizing the student residences, which were concentrated in a boarding house run by Upper Canada College English teacher Michael Barrett. At that time they cost king's a princely £319 a year, even though there were less than 14 students in the entire building! This was a controversial issue and Beaumont did not get his way at first. By the time of the meeting of October 28, however, he had managed to convince Council that the revenues needed for operating the residences should come from student fees alone, without additional King's College grants. Later, when Barrett decided to relinquish the residence, Beaumont and Gwynne convinced Council to place it under the control of the principal and one of the classical masters.[73]

Beaumont's cost-cutting extended throughout the college, even as far as the university president himself. On October 25 he voted against giving President John McCaul money to leave his home on the grounds of Upper Canada College so that he could rent a house off campus. He told McCaul to wait until the university finished constructing a new rent free house for him on its own ground.

Beaumont seems to have been fiscally very conservative in all areas of his life. Biographers claim that his favourite expression was "rich is he that neither has to beg nor borrow." He could afford to be complacent about money because he rarely had to make do without it. Despite the university's fiscal problems, for example, both he and Professor King saw their own salaries increase by £55. 11s. 2d. between 1848 and 1849 in recognition of their joint clinical lecturing at the Toronto General Hospital. All in all, Beaumont prospered over time from his association with King's College. His total college income for the period 1843 to 1849, which included his share of a thirty-shilling fee paid by students in the 1848-1849 academic year to attend his course, added up to a formidable £1898. 13s. 11d.

In 1849 Beaumont worked on Council towards more accountability from students and professors, yet at the same time he seemed to show a particular sympathy to the problems faced by part-time medical students. On February 17 he argued for more freedom for them outside college walls. As he put it, "It appears inexpedient, and perhaps illegal, to attempt to impose now on such students any restrictions as to their conduct without the walls of the university." He also had in mind students who visited the college during the day to hear just a few lectures. Occasional students such as these had long been permitted at the Rolph School, and King's College was now trying belatedly to catch up.

Why would Beaumont advocate this apparent loosening of the reins? Probably his attitude was born not so much from sympathy as expedience. Part-time medical students in mid-19th century Toronto had a reputation for rowdiness, bad language and rude behaviour and Beaumont was probably tired of being responsible for them. Live-in students, on the other hand, were restricted to their residences at night and were thereby more tightly controlled.

This is not to say, however, that Beaumont advocated a general loosening of control when it came to codes of conduct. On the contrary, it was precisely because the transitory nature of day students often led to their ignoring college rules on the pretext that they were not aware of the way the college was run — and hence could not be held accountable for their mistakes — that at the Council meeting February 24, Beaumont volunteered to lead a committee to supervise publication of the college's rules and statutes. Thereafter he made students sign the list of regulations when they were given their tickets to attend his lectures: no signature, no attendance!

In an effort at even-handedness, Beaumont offered his students certain compensations. Sometimes, for example, there were complaints that college money was not used in ways that were deemed appropriate by individual students. Beaumont proposed that all students be compelled to indicate to the Bursar at the time of payment of fees how they wanted their particular contribution to be used. The Bursar would then be required to make appropriate deposits in specific accounts.

In recognition of the fact that "sums of money have occasionally been given to various persons out of the Funds of the University, without the knowledge and consent of Council," Beaumont and Gwynne also tried to stop their colleagues from spending official funds without permission by proposing that the Bursar be responsible for all such payments. To their regret, the plan was deferred.

Beaumont's quest for accountability in the administration of King's College was timely in light of ever louder and more persistent demands for reform of the still largely Anglican college. Although a loyal member of the Church of England himself, Beaumont could see that change was inevitable, and it appears that his work on the Council was largely an effort to make the needed transitions as smooth as possible.

Many of these changes had their roots in religion and religious conflict. King's College was supposed to be non-denominational, but with powerful Anglicans in its government and administration this simply was not the case. Plans to reform the college had been proposed almost constantly since its formal opening in 1843, but they had never amounted to much. In 1843, for example, Baldwin introduced a university bill that would have affiliated King's College with the other three denominational colleges in the area: the Wesleyan Methodist Upper Canada Academy at Cobourg, founded in 1836, Queen's College, Kingston, established by the Presbyterians in 1841, and the Roman Catholic Regiopolis College, also in Kingston, which was founded by Bishop Alexander Macdonell in 1837. However, the plan failed when Baldwin's ministry collapsed in 1843.

In 1845 and 1846, two more attempts were made by Upper Canada Premier William Henry Draper to revive the Baldwin plan, but neither succeeded. The following year Receiver-General John A. Macdonald (1815-1891) tried to divide operating grants between King's College and the other three colleges. The King's College share was actually quite generous: the proposal was that it receive £3000 a year and the others £1500 each. Any extra funds would go into general education. Strachan rejected the proposal and again the government went out of office without reforming the college.

Much of the blame for the resistance to the secularization of King's College has to be laid squarely at the feet of Strachan. He was convinced that his task was to keep Upper Canada British. To that end, he steadfastly defended the Anglican monopoly of the Clergy Reserves, as well as Church of England domination in local politics. As long as he was in charge of King's College it would remain Anglican, and that's all there was to it!

Fortunately for the reformers, though, in 1848 Strachan finally resigned from the college presidency. Thereafter, change was rapid. In April 1849 the Baldwin University Bill was submitted to the Provincial Legislative Assembly. It asked for a non-denominational university in Upper Canada. King's College was quick to respond. On April 19, Beaumont formed a Council Committee to officially argue for amendments to the bill. On April 26 he wrote to Baldwin suggesting that the offices of University vice-chancellor and president be combined, and for election to the office by the Senate and Caput. He also said that election to the office should be held at short periodic intervals.

The Baldwin Bill was enacted in May 1849.[74] On 1 January 1850, King's College officially ceased to exist and became instead the non-denominational University of Toronto.

News of the formation of the University of Toronto left Strachan very unhappy. He was determined that the training of clergy not be left to chance and that Toronto should therefore have an Anglican university. He poured out his feelings in a letter to the province's Anglicans on 7 February 1850: "Deprived of her University, what is the Church to do? She now has no seminary in which to give a liberal education to her youth...I shall not rest satisfied till I have laboured to the utmost to restore the college under a holier and more perfect form."[75]

Now that the reformers had been given control of the university, however, they were not about to give it up. They had a lot of support, even among the province's Anglicans — including devout churchmen like

Beaumont. Strachan must have felt bitter indeed. What could he do now?

If it was impossible to restore King's College, Strachan decided, then he would have to form another Anglican college to replace it. On 10 April 1850 he left Toronto for England to obtain a charter for an Anglican university and to solicit funds for it. The charter would create a college "established on the clear and unequivocal principle" of adherence to the Church of England. Although at first unsuccessful, Strachan pleaded his case persistently and effectively and a charter was granted two years later.

Efforts in Toronto to raise funds for the new college went forward quickly. Strachan had donated money and land and many prominent local citizens quickly contributed to the cause, including Drs Hodder, Bovell and Burnside. Hodder and Bovell then found themselves agonizing all summer long over their options: should they stay in their old jobs, or should they join the new school?

By the fall of 1850 Hodder and Bovell had made up their minds and had organized a medical school for the new university, naming it the Upper Canada School of Medicine. As soon as Strachan returned from England in November they offered its presidency to him and Strachan was more than happy to accept. Advertisements for the school appeared in the *Toronto Patriot* newspaper, and it was formally opened by Strachan on November 7.

The medical faculty of Trinity University initially consisted of only six doctors: Hodder, Bovell, Henry Melville, Norman Bethune, William Hallowell and Francis Badgley. Hodder lectured in obstetrics and Bovell taught the institutes of medicine. Henry Melville (1816-1868), born in Barbados and educated at Edinburgh University, taught principles and practices of surgery every day at three o'clock, and hence was in direct competition with Beaumont. Norman Bethune (1822-1892) taught anatomy and physiology. He had actually studied liberal arts at King's College up to 1845, before he went to London and Edinburgh to get his medical education. William Hallowell (1814-1873) had studied medicine in England, France and Germany. He ended up teaching the early morning course in materia medica and therapeutics, including pharmaceutical chemistry. Francis Badgley taught the practice of medicine. He had been educated in Edinburgh and had had a thriving practice in Montreal.[76]

The Trinity Medical School began its life in an old jailhouse at the corner of King Street and Toronto Street and then moved to a large house on Spadina Avenue just north of Queen Street. On 30 April 1851 the cornerstone was laid for the Trinity University building. It was hoped that the medical school would eventually occupy the east side of the building, but this never happened.

In addition to teaching their first term of lectures and adding a summer school to their curricula along with the other faculty members, Hodder and Bovell launched a medical journal, the *Upper Canada Journal of Medical, Surgical and Physical Science*. This turned out to be too much of an undertaking for Hodder and Bovell to manage on their own, so King, O'Brien and Melville were co-opted and Beaumont also became one of the co-editors. He contributed several articles on his cataract cases at the Toronto Hospital between 1844-1851 to the first volume.

The first issue appeared in April 1851 and subscriptions were set at the inexpensive level of ten shillings a year. By contrast, the subscription to the rival Montreal *British American Journal of Medical and Physical Sciences* cost twice as much and the publishers complained that they could barely keep their heads above water at that price. Its low subscription rate may in fact have been one of the reasons for the eventual failure of the *Upper Canada Journal*. It survived until September 1854, when it printed its last issue.

Trinity College Medical School experienced difficulties from the start in meeting its operating costs. Within a year or two the lack of money had driven the school to accept a large number of non-Anglican students, which led to some heated exchanges with the Trinity University Council. In 1853, under heavy criticism, the college authorities published a list of requirements for their medical students, including the controversial "Rule Number 5," which insisted on belief in the tenets of the Anglican Church. "They will be required," it said, "before admission to the degree of M.B., to declare themselves bona fide members of the Church of England, and to subscribe [to] the Thirty Nine Articles of the 36th Canon." This demand constituted a serious threat to the medical school — for many of their best students belonged to other denominations — and it was vigorously challenged.

On 24 March, 1853, the *Toronto Globe* editorialized: "The most important enquiry is what the authority of the Queen in matters ecclesiastical, or the doctrine of the Thirty-Nine Articles, have to do with the education of young gentleman in the art of physicking her Majesty's liege subjects. Is there any necessary connection between setting a leg and setting the Church in order, between bringing babies into the world and baptismal regeneration? Could not young men be safely admitted within the walls of the college although they are followers of John Wesley or John Calvin?"

Would that the new school had listened! As it turned out, the criticism fell on deaf ears and soon the changes overtaking the educational system swept the Trinity Medical School away. In 1853 the University of Toronto stopped teaching law and medicine, only to have John A. Macdonald propose the revival of the medical faculty the following year. In the process, he implied that necessary faculty could be taken from Trinity University. The suggestion infuriated the Trinity Council, who gradually deprived its medical faculty of funding until the school finally collapsed in June 1856, when all its professors resigned. The cause of death was shortage of money and the inability to successfully combine medicine and religion. It was not to be reborn for another fifteen years.[77]

―― Chapter 8 ――

The Profession is Indebted

B y the close of 1850, confusion reigned supreme when it came to medical education in Toronto. There were three separate schools: the University of Toronto, the Toronto School of Medicine (Rolph's School) and the Trinity College Medical School, otherwise known as the Medical Faculty of the Church University or the Upper Canada School of Medicine. Each maintained its independence, operated its own facilities, offered its own courses and loudly proclaimed the inferiority of its two rivals. Yet despite these defamatory claims, students inevitably moved from one college to another, as did professors and demonstrators.

What about Toronto's institutions for the care of the sick? These were a little better organized. Foremost was the 107-bed Toronto General Hospital, which took up most of the city block between King, Adelaide, John and Peter Streets. It was dominated by the elderly Widmer, who was also one of the two leading figures at the Provincial Lunatic Asylum (John Scott was the other).There was the Toronto Eye Infirmary on the southwest corner of King and Church Streets, run by Dr. Samuel John Stratford (1798-1868), who had been educated in London and who had practised for many years in Woodstock. There were three maternity hospitals: the Toronto General Dispensary and Lying-In Hospital at the corner of Victoria and Richmond Streets, the Provincial Lying-In Hospital and

Vaccine Institute at 30 Richmond Street West and the Maternity Lying-In Hospital and General Dispensary at 36 Adelaide Street West (operated by the Rolph School). The House of Industry offered the medical services of Dr. Hodder. The Roman Catholic Orphan Asylum had Dr. Hayes.

What was Beaumont's role in all of this? By 1850 he had carved out an important and unique position in the arena of medical education, practice and administration in Toronto. In education he continued his successful course in surgery at the new University of Toronto and also gave lectures on surgery at the Toronto General Hospital.

In 1850, an honorary M.D. was conferred on him by the University of Toronto. As for medical practice, he treated patients both privately and at the hospital, where he was an attending physician. He was also visiting doctor for the nearby village of Springfield. Finally, Beaumont continued to serve as a member of the University of Toronto's administration and as a Commissioner on the Medical Board. The strain would eventually wear him down, but for now he was at the height of his career.

* * * *

Beaumont kept up his research and writing for the medical journals, both at home and abroad. He was not about to let his British colleagues forget about him. In 1850 he published a "Case of Disarticulation of the Left Condyle of the Lower Jaw" in the London *Medico-Chirurgical Transactions*. This article was based on his treatment of seven-year-old James McCugh, who was admitted to the Toronto General Hospital on 17 September 1849, his face distorted by a large (but painless) round tumour of the condyle of the mandible. The boy's appearance was heartrending. His teeth were deeply imbedded in the tumour, which kept him agape at all times and caused a constant dribbling of saliva from the corner of his mouth.

Beaumont consulted with Widmer, who was then the staff surgeon at the hospital. Through a curved incision from the ear to the corner of the mouth, Beaumont, with Widmer assisting, exposed the tumour. Having tied the facial artery to lessen bleeding from the tumour, he began to work on the condyle.

"I passed a strong ivory spatula," he wrote, "which using as a lever, I forced the tumour downwards from the malar bone."[78] Beaumont and Widmer cut the tumour from the facial muscles and removed it with its attached ligaments, cartilage and bone. They had successfully removed the tumour, but the operation had left "a large frightful hollow...where the tumour had been imbedded." The boy looked more dead than alive. "Three hare-lip pins were used to hold together the edges of the wound, with strips of adhesive plaster, over which cold water dressing was applied," Beaumont wrote. He gave James a large dose of opium to ease his pain and sent him back to his bed.

The post-operative course was complicated by wound infection with purulent discharge and by a salivary fistula, but two months after the operation the wound had healed, all discharge had stopped and Beaumont pronounced the boy "in perfect health." The tumour weighed 227 grams and comprised a "dense white cartilage, with numerous small particles of bone interspersed everywhere throughout the mass, as though it were undergoing ossification." A picture of the specimen appeared at the end of the article.

Shortly afterwards, Beaumont contributed a series of papers to the new *Upper Canada Journal of Medical, Surgical and Physical Science* in which he reported short case histories describing the most important of the cataract patients he had seen over the last few years at the Toronto Hospital.

Doctor Samuel Stratford, mentioned earlier in connection with the Toronto Eye Infirmary, was prominent in the later editing of this short-lived journal. At this point, Beaumont and Stratford were on good terms and Beaumont was more than willing to help advance Stratford's journal as a co-editor and by contributing papers to it. Their cordial relationship later soured, however, when they quarrelled over hospital visitation rights and Stratford published without permission one of Beaumont's clinical lectures on the treatment of false aneurysms.[79] Stratford and Beaumont carried on an ugly war of words in the journal over the next year which reflected badly on both of them.

* * * *

As Beaumont's research interests expanded, so did his administrative duties. In the spring of 1851, a government bill to incorporate the medical profession in Upper Canada included a clause that panicked many local doctors. The bill stated "that British Graduates and Members of British Colleges shall be excluded from the right of practicing in this Province, unless they undergo an examination in addition to that by which they obtained their British credentials."

Beaumont, his professional pride wounded, would have none of it and a majority of the other doctors in the city felt exactly the same way. Such a condition would reduce many of the doctors in Toronto to medical students again! On 7 May 1851, Beaumont and 28 others published their "entire dissent" to this proposal. In rejecting it, they declared, "we are confident that we shall carry the voice of a very large majority of the profession with us." They had reason to be confident. Their 29 signatures included those of most the city's prominent doctors, including King, Bovell, Widmer, Herrick and Richardson.

Those who did not sign included the doctors of the Toronto School of Medicine, including Rolph, Workman, Aikins, Langstaff and Morrison. The most likely reason for their boycott of the petition is that they thought the clause would hurt the competition more than it would them.

Fortunately, their dissent did not carry the day. The petition successfully intimidated the government and the examination idea was shelved.

This was good news for Beaumont. Indeed, the summer of 1851 saw happy times in his private life as well as his public life. His brother Edward came to visit him from England, and on 21 June 1851, his wife Mary Catherine gave birth to a son. Herbert Beaumont (1851-1923) was baptized by the Reverend Baldwin on October 19 at St. James' Cathedral and Edward served as one of the child's godfathers. William no doubt was glad to have a son. That November his daughter Charlotte celebrated her ninth birthday.

*   *   *   *

Towards the end of 1851 Beaumont returned to one of his favourite pastimes — the development of new medical instruments. This time it was an improved version of his fracture instrument, invented 20 years earlier. The older device had been designed for setting both broken legs and forearms.

The modification was intended specifically for the radius bone in the forearm.

It consisted of "an angular splint, made of gutta-percha, adapted to the bend of the elbow. To this is attached a bar of iron, which extends beyond the hand, and is then bent to a right angle. The latter portion has attached to it two axles, with ratchet wheels, for the purpose of making extension by means of cords attached to a leather cap laced to the wrist just above the joint. In addition, there are two small splints adapted to the anterior and posterior part of the forearm."

This sounds more complicated than it really is. In essence, the patient placed his broken arm in the instrument, whose tightened cords would then exert a steady pull on the limb. This held the broken long bone in its natural alignment and prevented the arm muscles from deforming it during healing. The patient's arm was wrapped with bandages "to protect the skin from any painful pressure" and if the traction made the skin beneath the leather cap painful, it could be reduced by "throwing the catch out of the teeth of the ratchet-wheel, and allowing the angle to revolve backwards."

Beaumont used his instrument in the Toronto Hospital with great results. It was also successfully adopted by other surgeons, whose testimonials he reproduced in a published article.[80] Doctor J.W. Warren called it a "very efficient apparatus" and praised "Professor Beaumont, of Toronto, to whom the profession is indebted for the invention of many ingenious surgical instruments, some of which have been for a long time in use at our Hospital."

Beaumont hoped he could soon use the device for more than fractures of the radius. With luck, he could use it on the other bone of the forearm, the ulna, or even on the humerus in the upper arm.

* * * *

In 1852 a drastic change took place at the Medical Board when, at Rolph's urging, Governor General James Bruce Elgin (1811-1863) supplemented the membership with a group of Toronto School of Medicine graduates, including Rolph himself, Workman, Aikins and Morrison, thereby more than tripling the size of the Board. Now at least Rolph could no longer criticize the Board for its discrimination against his candidates, since it was packed full of them. Equally, the former Board members could no longer complain about being overworked.

The changes did not free Beaumont from administrative duties, however. Far from it. In July he attended a series of meetings at the Toronto Mechanics' Institute designed to incorporate the medical profession in Upper Canada. The idea behind these meetings came from Widmer, who had evidently hoped to defeat Rolph's reform of the Board by establishing an incorporated medical profession that would supersede it. This plan was heavily criticized by Rolph's school graduates, including Workman, who bitterly accused Widmer of "acting cat's paw for the Tories."[81]

Widmer himself was absent from the meetings because of illness. However, all his friends, including Beaumont, were there. They vigorously debated the text of a proposed "Act to Incorporate the Medical Profession in Upper Canada." This Act was published in the September edition of the *Upper Canada Journal of Medical, Surgical and Physical Sciences*. It named Beaumont as one of the members of a "College of Physicians and Surgeons of Upper Canada" which would have a separate Board of Governors to regulate medical licences.

Just when it began to look as though Rolph's packed Medical Board would be eased out of office, he and others were able to scuttle the proposal with vigorous lobbying efforts of their own. Incorporation of the profession remained as elusive as ever, a casualty of radical opposition groups and feuding between medical institutions.[82]

Beaumont must have been highly dissatisfied with this failure, but with all his administrative duties he had little time to brood. One of his most onerous tasks was serving on the various governing bodies of the University of Toronto. The work was important, but much of it involved tedious meetings that often had little to do with his real love, medicine. Even so, he continued to attend faithfully and to take an active role in the discussions.

The University Senate meeting of 3 August, 1852 was typical. Beaumont and other members were bogged down in a long discussion about the creation of two new professorships at the college: the Chair of Mineralogy and Geology and the Chair of Natural History. Beaumont tried to delay their establishment by questioning the legal powers of the Caput, the Visitation Committee and the other groups that had proposed the chairs in the first place. Ever true to his fiscal conservatism, he also questioned any presumed right to attach salaries to the chairs. Vigorous discussion ensued. Although the University President was with him,

Beaumont lost the debate and the motion to create the two chairs was carried. He did manage, however, to persuade the Senate to attach to the resolution a statement describing his doubts, which would be seen by the Governor General when he read the resolution.

Beaumont was back at the Senate the very next day, August 4, lobbying for funds for a new medical building. Beaumont got what he wanted and retired from the meeting.

In the fall of 1852 Beaumont continued to preach fiscal restraint and government accountability. (His knack for spotting detail in financial records was astounding. In the course of looking over the university's account books, for example, local auditors made several entries and corrections. Beaumont and one of his colleagues, Professor Skeffington Connor, subsequently found an error in the auditors' calculations, corrected the mistake and told the auditors to leave the books alone!) He convinced the Senate to inform the Provincial Secretary of all university laws, statutes and rules, and during a later meeting he helped to edit the text of a new University Bill soon to be submitted to the government. A few weeks later he appointed a committee to "investigate into the duties and salaries of Professors, and general management of the University." Finally, at the December 14 Senate meeting he sponsored candidates for the new Chair of Civil Engineering at the University of Toronto. Beaumont recommended his old friend George Herrick for the post over N. Marshall and F.W. Cumberland.

It was a hectic life and the strain on Beaumont was beginning to tell. He was involved in so many medical programmes and sitting on so many boards and committees that he began to show signs of burnout as he raced around between the university, various hospitals and his private patients. There simply were never enough hours in the day.

Public criticism levelled against the University of Toronto and the General Hospital added to the strain. At the university there was a great deal of unhappiness with an educational system that had no religious foundation, but no one could agree on how to restore the element of faith, or indeed which denomination to base it on. And over at the hospital crippling shortages of money and qualified practitioners were making it very difficult to keep the place running.

On 19 February 1853, Beaumont's old friend Widmer was installed as University Chancellor but, as it turned out, even this influential colleague could not protect Beaumont from changes that were sweeping in.

In the Surrogate Court of the
County of York

In the Goods of William Rawlins Beaumont
deceased

Inventory of Personal Estate	Value
Proceeds of Life Policy in the Scottish Provincial Assurance	$2335.00
Mortgage on Wellington St. house made by John Ginty	2000.00
Deposit in Bank of British North America	400.00
Interest thereon at 4% from the 5th of March 1875 to 5 Nov 1875	10.66
Deposit (current account) in Bank of B.N.A.	57.61
Plate (silver)	145.00
Surgical Instruments	59.00
Books (Surgical & miscellaneous)	138.00
Carpenters tools	23.00
Furniture	142.00
Clothing	51.00
	$5461.27

Beaumont's goods at death, 1875. (Archives of Ontario.)

Beaumont's Will. (Archives of Ontario.)

On March 3, *McKenzie's Weekly Message* charged that members of the provincial government were trying to "abolish the faculties of Law and Medicine" at the University of Toronto with the 1853 Hincks Act. This Act was an effort by Prime Minister Sir Francis Hincks to deal with the many critics of the "godless university" that had sprung up after the secularization of King's College. Now that the various religious denominations each had their own colleges, it asked, what was the proper role for the University of Toronto? The Anglicans had Trinity, the Methodists had Victoria, the Presbyterians had Queen's and the Roman Catholics had Regiopolis. What more could a secular college add?

The idea behind the Hincks Act was to convert the University of Toronto into an examining college only, with actual instruction being carried out at the various religious colleges, which would then be affiliated with the University of Toronto, supporting it through their teaching faculties. But it did not happen this way. University College, which lost the right to teach law and medicine under the Act, instead became a small arts college supported mainly by low church Anglicans suspicious of Trinity and Presbyterians distrustful of Queen's. It was not until 1860, when a large University College building was erected, that the university began to grow again. This growth was accelerated seven years later when, under Confederation, the University of Toronto was made the provincial university of Ontario.

As for Hincks, his government collapsed in 1854, the victim of growing sectional rivalries, clergy reserve controversies and railroad corruption.

Who was behind the Hincks Act? Certainly none of the doctors at the University of Toronto, who obviously had the most to lose by the medical school's abolition. And Trinity Medical School had enough problems of its own. By 1853 it was sliding inevitably towards chaos, arguing over finances and religious tests. That left the Toronto School of Medicine. What was Rolph up to during all the turmoil?

The answer, as it turns out, is quite a lot. Rolph was an important and influential member of the Hincks government. He would have a great deal to gain if the University of Toronto stopped teaching medicine. Everyone could see that Trinity was in decline. If Beaumont's school could be shut down too, the Toronto School of Medicine would reign supreme. Even if Trinity survived it would be a lot easier to compete against one school than two. Moreover, Rolph argued, why should medical students be trained at public expense? After all, they were in training for a lucrative profession and would certainly be well paid when they got out of school.

Rolph's criticisms carried a lot of weight, particularly when the general public was already angry over the non-denominational nature of the University of Toronto. Logical and persuasive as such arguments sound, however, hearsay had it that there was something a lot more sinister afoot. According to University Librarian William Stewart Wallace (1884-1970), who wrote the history of the University of Toronto, it was widely rumoured that Rolph told Hincks he would support the government's beloved Grand Trunk Railroad if Hincks would shut down the medical school at the University of Toronto. The truth may never be known. Trinity College's Dean, Walter Bayne Geikie (1830-1917), for example, later claimed that it was utter nonsense. Nevertheless, it is clear that Rolph saw the University of Toronto as a stumbling block to his own aspirations and bitterly resented its lengthy domination of local medical education and administration.

In any event, Rolph or no Rolph, the medical faculty of the University of Toronto was out of business by the end of 1853. The defeat hit Beaumont particularly hard. He lost not only his position as lecturer in surgery, which he had held for 10 years, but also his job as Dean of the Medical School. At least he still had his private practice and his work as physician to the Toronto General Hospital. Unfortunately, however, the Toronto General Hospital was beginning to experience troubles of its own.

── Chapter 9 ──
He should have Dr. Beaumont

The Toronto General Hospital was the largest hospital in the city and the one where the majority of clinical research was done. It was, therefore, closely monitored by staff, patients and the general public. Sadly, even before the medical faculty of the University of Toronto became defunct, facilities had already begun to fall into disrepair at the hospital and few efforts were being made to keep up with the most recent advances in medicine and surgery. In 1853 the profession and the general public both reexamined the hospital — and neither liked what it saw.

Years of chronic underfunding lay at the root of the hospital's troubles. No one was willing to provide the funds for the expansion and new equipment necessary for meeting the needs of a growing population of 30 000 souls, a population that just nine years earlier had been a mere 18 000.

In February 1853, a hard-hitting editorial appeared edition in the *Upper Canada Journal of Medical, Surgical and Physical Science*. Largely the work of Stratford, it had very little to say about the hospital that was positive, preferring instead to catalogue its faults, condemn its trustees and call for change.

"The condition of the present Hospital building is extremely bad, both old and inefficient," it charged, "and although capable of containing 75 beds, it is entirely without due and necessary ventilation, while there is no chance of properly heating the building...besides which the building leaks extremely, and the toute ensemble is a perfect picture of ruin and decay, that ill accords with the rapid progress of the good city of Toronto."

The journal complained that the hospital was bad not only for patients, but for doctors too. Beaumont must have read these lines sympathetically, and perhaps they were particularly intended for his attention: "To the Medical Officer it is a constant source of annoyance, perhaps he has treated the patient with the most consummate skill and science, and he naturally expects to find the legitimate result of his appropriate treatment, but as the deadly poison received into the patient's constitution [from the Hospital's foul air] so modifies the result, that it is anything but what it was intended, and instead of obtaining a cure, he has to combat a far worse malady at an enormous disadvantage."

How often had Beaumont seen his work ruined by wound infection!

"The Medical Officers," the article said, "might divide their duties as Surgeon and Physician. The duties of these Medical Officers should be to attend the Hospital punctually at the hour of 12 o'clock, according to their turns of duty. Each should be obliged to inscribe his name and the hour of his arrival, in a book kept for the purpose, at the Hospital, and this should be laid before the Board at their monthly meeting; if the Hospital rule has not been punctually attended to, and no sufficient excuse offered for absence or delay, due punishment should follow; for it must be remembered that time is of vital importance to the Medical Student, when he has numerous lectures to attend to."

Unfortunately, a busy schedule meant that Beaumont himself was often late at the hospital and was not always on hand when students asked for him. This was to become an important issue when he was placed "on trial" at the trustees' investigations two years later.

The article's revelations aroused much comment in professional circles, but the complaints were also clearly heard by the general public as well. It was not long before newspaper editors read the articles, made their own investigations, and then embellished them with pieces of their own. The most scathing criticism appeared in the 22 March 1853 edition of the *Semi-Weekly Leader*.

"The hospital building is almost entirely destitute of the conveniences which it ought to possess," it charged. It went on to catalogue the deficiencies of the hospital, which extended from the basement to the roof. The lack of ventilation, for example, led to "a foulness of the air extremely dangerous to the patients, medical officers, students, attendants and others whose duty is frequently to visit the wards." The odour permeated the entire building, leaving it "almost impossible for a patient to escape this noxious influence as is shown by the constant attacks of erysipelas and...other complaints that indiscriminately affect them after residing a short time in the hospital."

The lack of adequate plumbing and toilets was a public disgrace. "There is not a water closet in the whole building nor within at least eighty yards [73 metres] of it. There is no bathhouse in the building unless one old tin concern can be dignified with that name. To reach this the patient has to wander through the basement to a rickety temporary washhouse, otherwise the solitary tin bath may be hauled up two pairs of stairs by main force and the water carried after it in pails which at least has the advantage of security against scalding the patient as the water has ample time to cool off."

And the bedding? Most of the patients' blankets "would be rejected by any spirited stableboy if offered as a horse rug. Except for a dozen sent by the mayor during the last cholera epidemic, not a new blanket has entered the institution in the last six years." In the lower wards, conditions were truly pitiful: "The ceilings are mottled with damp, as water percolated through the upper floors in washing where the floors were worn and broken, and the floor in proximity to the stove has holes three inches [8 centimetres] wide and a foot or two [30 to 60 centimetres] long."

Beaumont operated under particularly trying conditions. There was no operating room. Instead, surgery was performed in the wards or in a corridor, "the cries of the patient being heard by all the invalids no matter how injurious such a disturbance may be to them."

The *Leader* was disgusted with the filth and mess. The temptation was to blame the staff, but the newspaper found that their lot was just as bad. "The Matron is stored away in a sort of cell of most scant dimensions in the basement and that dreary solitary underground room serves her for eating, sleeping and other purposes," it wrote. "The Resident Physician and Surgeon receive the munificent sum of 100 pounds a year [Beaumont's lectures at the hospital were gratis] and an unfurnished room without board or servant for unremitting attention to from sixty to seventy patients."

Clearly radical changes were necessary, including new governors and new facilities. "The time has arrived when some reform in the management of this Provincial Institution is imperatively required," the newspaper wrote, presenting an elaborate list of demands. Among them was a "theatre for surgical operations" and a reception room for new patients. Beaumont would have been happy to get the operating theatre, but there was little hope of immediate action. All the city's medical institutions were calling for change. Reform would have to wait for another day.

Thus the appalling conditions at the Toronto Hospital continued through 1853. The only change saw Beaumont and six other physicians formally appointed as the "hospital staff" by the trustees. Forced to work cheek by jowl in the cramped wards, they were supervised by Beaumont's friend Widmer, who was the consulting physician and surgeon and a member of the Board of Trustees, and indeed, for all the hardships, they worked well together. In fact, the very shortage of material may have been one of the spurs that prompted Beaumont to improvise more instruments of his own.

In the end, however, his dissatisfaction with conditions finally did erupt into a full scale brawl with Stratford. The whole unhappy mess started on 16 January 1854, with Beaumont's lecture on "false aneurisms" to his students.[83] This lecture was based on his experience with a 20-year-old patient named Joseph Sterves, who had been stabbed in the neck with a large knife.

A doctor had stopped the bleeding by applying a compress and bandages, but it had started again the next day it after the patient sneezed, and he had been brought to Beaumont for treatment. Beaumont had sewn the wound and it looked as if Sterves had been saved from certain death. A day later, however, a "small beating tumour" had started to form in the wound and had steadily increased until it was the size of a hen's egg. This was the false aneurysm of Beaumont's lecture to his students. It had been caused by an escape of blood from the small wound in the wall of the carotid artery. The surrounding tissues had prevented the collection of blood from spreading. The students listened with their stethoscopes to the pulsating turbulence in the aneurysm. They heard the "rush in the tumour produced by the constant whirl of arterial blood as it enters, takes its course through the tumour, and finds an exit again into the blood vessels."

Beaumont decided treatment should consist of Valsalva's method, which involved "frequent small bleedings and a strict diet, with the careful use of the digitalis." If that failed, he planned to cut the tumour out, placing a ligature above and below the wound made in the artery. This was the operation that had been perfected by George James Guthrie (1785-1856), an army surgeon who had practised surgery at the Battle of Waterloo in 1815. During campaigns in Spain and France he had seen many traumatic aneurysms and was recognized as the foremost authority on battle surgery in the early nineteenth century. As it turned out, however, an operation was not needed, because healing of the aneurysm took place during Beaumont's administration of the Valsalva regime[84] and after five months "the tumour was no longer visible."[85]

Beaumont had intended to publish this case in the pages of the *Lancet* where his English friends and colleagues could see it. Unfortunately, one of the students at Beaumont's lecture that day had been listening with much more than his usual attention — he had written down almost everything Beaumont had said. To Beaumont's surprise he received a letter from Stratford a few days later asking permission to publish the student's version in the *Upper Canada Journal of Medical, Surgical and Physical Science*.

Beaumont was careful not to turn Stratford down directly. Instead, he wrote back saying that he "could not consent to the publication of the Clinical Lecture on Traumatic Carotid Aneurism from notes taken by a student, unless such notes and the proof should first be corrected by Dr. Beaumont, and which he was willing to do, if such notes were tolerably accurate."[86]

Stratford was delighted. He immediately ordered the paper to be published, wrote a lengthy postscript explaining the paper's format, and sent Beaumont a copy of the proofs for correction. Then things went wrong.

Beaumont wrote back to Stratford, complaining that the proofs were flawed. As he put it, "the proof which you have sent me contains a great deal which I did not say, and gives very incorrectly and imperfectly parts of the lecture, as well as the quotations from Guthrie." He was also unhappy about the postscript that Stratford had added, which was less an explanation than a litany of complaints against Beaumont. It pointed out that his novel method of treatment was not to be seen in the standard textbooks, that Guthrie had never recommended what Beaumont was doing and that Beaumont had denied Stratford access to the book he had quoted from in class. Finally, Stratford complained that he had not seen the patient himself because Beaumont had insisted on being in attendance when he did so, and "although we daily waited upon Dr. Beaumont's arrival, we have not had an opportunity of seeing the case in question. In saying this much we do not wish to make any unkind remarks upon the irregular way in which Dr. Beaumont attends at the hospital. Nevertheless we cannot fail to offer our modicum of praise for the zeal and industry with which we see that Dr. Hodder, Aikins and some other gentlemen attend to their hospital duties."[87]

Beaumont was hardly likely to consent to a gratuitous comment like that appearing in print. He politely told Stratford to forget it and sent his manuscript off to the *Lancet*. But by now it was too late. Stratford was either unable or unwilling to stop the proofs and the article appeared in the March 1854 edition of the journal.

Beaumont was outraged. He immediately called a special meeting of the officers of the hospital and poured out his side of the whole sorry story. The paper needed corrections, he argued, and should never have been published in that form; moreover, the postscript had no business being there in the first place. Hodder was quick to come to Beaumont's defence regarding his colleague's reputation for tardiness. Widmer listened with sympathy and wrote an angry letter on March 10 to Stratford demanding that the next issue of the journal correct the mistakes and include a statement of the editor's disappointment and regret. Stratford complied, but added a sullen note saying that if Beaumont wanted so much to correct the paper, why couldn't he have done it before it was published? Furthermore, why had Hodder gone to so much trouble to defend Beaumont's irregular hospital attendance when he had earlier complained about it himself? "Indeed this is a curious world we live in, not inconsistent, certainly!!" Stratford commented bitterly.

The break was complete. Beaumont denied Stratford hospital visiting privileges and sent a letter describing Stratford's unprofessional conduct to the *Lancet*. It was apparently so inflammatory that the Lancet, which had published much of Beaumont's other work, refused to print it. Shortly after that, the *Upper Canada Journal of Medical, Surgical and Physical Science* collapsed, a victim of tight budgets and squabbling doctors.

There is an ironic coda to this tale. Beaumont's case study, which was supposedly so inaccurate and unworthy of publication, was eventually printed in at least three places. The first was Stratford's journal, the second was the July 29, 1854, edition of the *Lancet* and the third was the January 1855 *Retrospect of Practical Medicine and Surgery*, the journal of the Leeds Medical School obstetrics lecturer W. Braithwaite — not bad exposure for a students' record of a clinical lecture!

While Beaumont and Stratford were feuding in the medical journals, conditions at the Toronto hospital were going from bad to worse. In March 1855 the situation reached a crisis when the *Toronto Colonist* published a scathing letter from an anonymous medical student criticizing the hospital conditions and charging that Trinity students were being given preference over students from the Rolph school. He also complained that visiting physicians were ignoring students' needs. Beaumont must have felt that this last criticism was intended particularly for him. After all, he still had a problem with punctuality.

A new hospital had in fact been built on Gerrard Street, but it had not yet been occupied and the hospital trustees decided that an investigation into the various charges was appropriate. It began with their meeting on March 29 and lasted three days.[88]

The crowded boardroom first heard Secretary J.W. Brent read the letter, which began with a stinging indictment of the hospital and its staff. It accused the orderlies and nurses of routinely mistreating patients, particularly those of other races, citing as an example an orderly named Burns who had been fined a pound by the police for his cruelty to a black patient.

"This is not a solitary or isolated instance of this man's conduct," the letter read. "His cruelty and ruthlessness are proverbial among students."

The police had hoped Burns would be fired, but he had remained on staff. As for the nurses, one was cited as having "a heart as callous and impervious to the appeals of common humanity [as Burns]. Her coarseness, insolence and rudeness are too notorious to every observer to need comment."

The doctors, according to the letter, were no better than the support staff. House surgeon Edward Clarke was accused of refusing to allow a medical student to extract an indigent man's tooth, insisting instead that the patient pay a regular dentist to do the job. The poverty-stricken individual simply could not afford this and was forced to do without dental care. "Is this fact to go abroad, that in the 'Toronto General Hospital' a poor man cannot have a tooth extracted?" the author demanded. "It would be a disgrace to our city."

The hospital's appearance was also the target of criticism. "It is so filthy, that it is best known among those who walk the wards by the appellation of the 'Lousy Hospital'; and it is only mentioned to sneer and ridicule it as a fountain of moral pollution. The time spent by the student is considered worse than squandered; no remuneration is received to compensate for the loss of the £2, much less their time; and were it not that our colleges demand a twelve month's hospital attendance, few, if any, students would visit it, but to learn how much misery and disease are augmented within its walls."

The letter concluded by threatening to disclose more horrors to the public in the future if these problems were not corrected immediately.

The reading caused an outcry at the meeting, forcing the Trustees to defend themselves as best they could. The author was identified as a student named James Dixon and he was brought forward for questioning. During their interrogation, the Trustees were able to expose the fact that Dixon was wanting himself: he had studied medicine for only eight months and he had never had a hospital ticket authorizing him to study on the wards. Meanwhile Widmer pleaded poverty as the reason for lack of equipment at the hospital. Next, "counter" letters were produced, one from Hospital Secretary Brent, the other from an anonymous "Veritas." They flatly denied Dixon's claims.

Beaumont sat and listened to it all. At first, some of the testimony that he heard was even gratifying. It was reported, for example, that the "cruel nurse" Mrs. Donnelly (who was anything but cruel to his way of thinking) had taken the parents of a young boy suffering from a fistula to one side and had told them "to get Dr. Hodder or Dr. Beaumont to operate upon him...he would die in the Hospital if left under Dr. Aikins' care." But it was not long, however, before criticism devolved onto Beaumont as well.

A senior medical student, John Lennon, who had been studying at Rolph's school, complained that Beaumont and the other doctors were never at the hospital during their scheduled hours. "I have not had the privilege of walking with them," he said. "Dr. Beaumont will not come sometimes until three o'clock. It is not once in six weeks that I meet with them, and yet I must come up here and wait my hour from twelve to one o'clock, in order to get my ticket certified, or if I don't, I cannot graduate at College. I don't know why Dr. Herrick or Dr. Beaumont don't attend." Lennon charged that the Trustees had known of this problem for a long time but had done nothing about it. "The subject was brought under Dr. Widmer's notice," he said, but "Dr. Beaumont said he would attend when he liked."

Suddenly things were looking decidedly ominous. Then Hodder stepped in to protect his friend. He pointed out that when he had been sick during the past winter and had been unable to make his rounds at the hospital, "he had got Dr. Beaumont or Dr. Bovell to see his patients for him." Beaumont was able to breathe a sigh of relief, and the rest of the day's testimony passed without incident. He went home content when the meeting adjourned at six o"clock.

The inquiry resumed at noon the next day. Beaumont saw himself alternately condemned and praised. The first charge he had to defend was an accusation by Ogden of the use of "immoral language," an issue over which the two had already crossed swords. Beaumont pointed out that "immoral language" was a relative term and suggested that Ogden repeat the offending words if he wanted to make a case. Initially Ogden balked. After all, there were ladies in the room and coarse language in front of ladies constituted a serious breach of etiquette in the Canada of 1855. But that didn't stop the discussion. The trustees sent all the ladies out of the room and Ogden repeated the words, asking Beaumont if he was satisfied. "He might at least have spared his audience, if he had no regard for his own feelings," Ogden complained.

On the plus side, Beaumont did get some support that day from a student who defended him against the charge of not doing enough work at the hospital. "It struck me as being very singular," he said, "that although Dr. Telfer and Dr. Beaumont had been known as Hospital attendants for a length of time, that it rarely happened that a fair share of surgical practice fell into their hands. I thought that they did not get their share of surgical practice and my impression was that they would have taken it if they could have gotten it." The witness tried to portray Beaumont as being unavailable only because he was being unfairly deprived of his share of patients. Once again Beaumont was off the hook.

The hearing wound up the next day. This time Beaumont faced a more serious opponent: William Aikins. Lennon asked Aikins if he knew about Herrick and Beaumont skipping their hospital rounds. Aikins was happy to cooperate. His attack was bitter and sustained: "The students complained of Dr. Herrick's non-performance of duty, and of Dr. Beaumont's coming at such hours as prevented them going the rounds with him to see his patients, and of Dr. Beaumont's stating that he would visit his patients at whatever hour suited himself best."

Aikins then proceeded to charge that Beaumont discriminated against him: "In several operations of Dr. Beaumont, I have not been consulted, while other medical men, not belonging to the Institution, have been consulted," he complained.

Once again one of Beaumont's friends intervened. A former student named Richardson said the reason Beaumont did not come on time was because recently he was seeing patients affected with aneurysms who could not be disturbed by noisy medical students. Aikins backtracked, admitting that while Beaumont was tardy, it had to be admitted that his patients were never neglected. But he also pointed out that the problem had been going on since long before the aneurysm cases: "It has been a complaint for four or five years to my certain knowledge."

Richardson continued to defend Beaumont, emphasizing the importance of quiet for these patients and adding that in contrast Stratford had taken his Toronto School of Medicine students into the ward and disturbed them.

The meeting continued with the reading of a letter from Beaumont and four other doctors that condemned Dixon and called his attack in the *Daily Colonist* "a tissue of malicious falsehoods." They suggested instead that "the greatest credit is due to Dr. Clarke, the resident medical officer, for the general good order and cleanliness of the Hospital, and also for the zeal, attention and ability which he has, for so many years, shown in the discharge of his onerous and frequently unpleasant professional duties. With regard to the orderly, Burns, and the nurse alluded to, we desire to say we have never observed anything approaching to cruelty on their parts, and we believe them both to be steady, honest, and well deserving servants of the Institution."

Beaumont's defence seemed to be gaining acceptance, but Widmer decided nevertheless to call upon Beaumont to take the stand and answer the charges against him. In response, Beaumont informed the assembly that, being technically out of a job (by now it had been two years since the University of Toronto had laid him off), he could no longer be counted upon to teach medical students. He gently reminded his audience of a critical difference between himself and surgeons like Clarke and others, a difference that had apparently been forgotten in the heat of all these arguments. "They receive fees from the students for their instruction and have a claim upon their attendance. Here we do our duty gratuitously, and the public must know that whenever duty is done gratuitously a great deal of allowance must be made. The Trustees did not say I should attend regularly at noon. I have however attended regularly so far as regards my patients. When in the Toronto University I did attend regularly every day but it is different now. I do not consider, however, that the students have the slightest claim upon me for instruction."

This speech took a lot of steam out of the protestors. How could they complain about someone who was working for them for free?

Unfortunately, however, Beaumont did not stop there. Convinced that Toronto School of Medicine graduates were inferior to begin with, and probably still unhappy over Rolph's role in the scuttling of his job at the University of Toronto, he concluded his speech by attacking the professional competence of Aikins and his colleague Henry Hover Wright, Rolph School instructors both.

"Every man must begin to operate," Beaumont said, "but those are best qualified to begin who have seen operations performed, and Dr. Aikins and Dr. Wright I must say have not had opportunities of seeing a great many surgical operations performed."

Aikins was furious. "When you make a statement against my professional ability," he snapped, "I think you ought to be able to substantiate every word you say."

Beaumont pushed on, reminding the audience that Wright and Aikins had been trained locally — and therefore simply could not have seen as many operations as those surgeons who had been trained in the United States or England. "There is a certain responsibility involved in taking part in operations which I should not desire to share, unless with persons whom I know to be in the habit of operating. I should not greatly desire to assist in an operation performed either by Dr. Aikins or by Dr. Wright. I should not desire to do so." Aikins and Wright should be demoted to hospital assistants, he advised...they were too inexperienced to handle greater responsibility.

The question may be asked, why did Beaumont exhibit such enduring hostility? The answer may well lie in the fact that Aikins had written earlier to Rolph complaining of improper behaviour on Beaumont's part. According to Aikins, Beaumont examined one of his own medical students from the university and insisted on giving him a pass. Students from Rolph's School subsequently complained about the apparent favouritism to the Board chairman, Widmer, who merely responded that Beaumont was quite capable of examining his own students. Aikins, infuriated, protested Beaumont's conduct in a newspaper editorial entitled "Good Doctors and Safe People," making Beaumont look autocratic, heavy handed and unfair.

Whatever the reasons for Beaumont's vitriol, both Aikins and Wright, for their part, were outraged by the scathing assessment of their abilities. A few weeks later they had ample reason to be even more unhappy.

The trustees ended the public inquiry on March 31 and retired to consider the matter in private. Two weeks later, on April 14, the Hospital Board sent the two doctors letters informing them their services as medical officers were no longer required.

Aikins and Wright were not about to give up without a fight. They immediately appealed the suspension to the Provincial Legislature, which ruled early in 1856 that, since the Board had not been unanimous in its decision, they had to be given their jobs back. They returned to the hospital in triumph, satisfied with the decision — and bitterly angry with Beaumont. Aikins in particular would nurse a long-standing grudge against him and plan a later revenge.

And what happened to the hospital reforms in all of this? Not much, though the press continued with its criticisms.

A chronicle from May 1855 repeats familiar complaints: "the floors, walls, and ward appurtenances are extremely filthy; the ubiquitous patients swarming with vermin; no ablutions, no baths." Nurses and orderlies were cruel and physicians did not come to the hospital on time. Even Beaumont "came at no appointed hour; so that the élèves [students] could not participate in the benefits anticipated in selecting this institution for the study of disease."

By now, however, the public was getting tired of the familiar litany of protests and instead was looking toward the opening of the new Toronto General Hospital. This took place the following year in 1856. The old building was handed back to the government and was used as office space until it's demolition six years later. The city of Toronto had moved into a new era of medical care.

—— Chapter 10 ——
New Hospitals and New Surgeons

The new Toronto General Hospital, constructed in the spring of 1854 on the north side of Gerrard Street between Sackville and Sumach Streets, opened its doors to the general public on 1 October 1856, when 12 patients were transferred there from the old hospital.

It provided much better facilities than the old one on King Street West and John Street. To begin with, it had a modern operating theatre, which must have been a great joy to Beaumont. There were also several baths, water closets and washrooms and the building was liberally sprinkled with air vents and flues to ensure adequate supplies of fresh air.

Unfortunately, although the building itself was new, all the grievances and grudges from the old building were transferred with the staff.

Around the beginning of 1856, Aikins began to keep a private diary of what he saw as Beaumont's misconduct. He found a lot to record over the next few months. In January 1856 he recorded the following: "1. Ligature of the vein as well as the artery. 2. The polyp case and forceps. 3. Lithotomy cases. 4. Fistula of perineum — operation unsuccessful — death. 5. The case of empyema — treated as psoas abscess — dislocation of shoulder — the ignorance and cruelty."[89]

By June 30, Aikins had written much more and he felt he now had evidence of Beaumont's surgical incompetence. Not only did he continue to arrive late at the hospital, but on occasion he had even shown signs of intoxication. Here is Aikins' account: "Beaumont comes at 1/4 afternoon, five minutes later went slying along to visit a lithotomy case — I followed, he saw me and shut the door in my face. I opened it and went in — he was not [unreadable] enough to speak — order the mother and nurse not to allow anyone to see him except Dr. Widmer or Dr. Clark."[90]

Aikins told other doctors at the hospital about Beaumont's behaviour, but as long as Widmer was in charge he had to be careful. Besides, who would believe him? His humiliation in front of the Trustees' investigation had been seen by the entire city.

Fortunately for Beaumont, Aikins's private notes were not read or made public until long after they had both died. The lithotomy case, on the other hand, alluded to in Aikins's descriptions of Beaumont's odd behaviour was indeed to become well known, for it provided the material for his next series of publications.

Beaumont's "Clinical Lecture on the Several Forms of Lithotomy" was formally delivered at the Toronto General Hospital during the winter of 1855-1856, but he delayed publishing it, perhaps because his experience with Stratford had taught him to be more careful. It appeared in the *Lancet* in January 1857 and then a synopsis was published in the *Retrospect of Practical Medicine and Surgery*.

Lithotomy, the removal of a stone from the urinary bladder, is one of the oldest surgical operations, singled out by Hippocrates long ago as one of the operations that should be performed only by specialists. Beaumont began his article by showing considerable talent as a medical historian in reviewing the eight major lithotomy techniques known up to his time. These ranged from the rough scalpel and hook method of Celsus in the first century A.D. to the recto- urethral operation performed "about eight months ago" at Beaumont's alma mater, St. Batholomew's Hospital in London.

Beaumont then described what he thought was a unique case involving the first lithotomy patient "into whose bladder a glass catheter has been passed." Richard Nichols, a 26-year-old Brampton man, had been admitted into Toronto General Hospital on 8 November 1855. He had been using an elastic catheter to empty his bladder for over a year, but when a glass-blower came to town, he had had the "misfortune to conceive the idea of a glass catheter, and to get one made," Beaumont wrote. Not surprisingly, it broke in his bladder and Nichols came to the hospital the next day in great pain.

Beaumont introduced a no. 11 silver catheter into the urethra to make sure the glass fragments would not become trapped there. To remove the glass he used a large curved staff, grooved on its convex side. The groove provided a channel through which he could introduce a modified pair of "polypus forceps, the blades of which I had grooved lengthwise, and lined with leather, the better to hold the glass, and guard against its breaking when grasped by the forceps."

After a dozen attempts, he managed to grab the catheter by its end and worked it out of the bladder. The operation was difficult, but eventually successful.

Nichols recovered quickly. The next day, the temporary gum-elastic catheter Beaumont had inserted was removed and "the urine now passed freely through the urethra...He felt well, his appetite was good, and his pulse 84." Beaumont continued to monitor Nichols's pulse over the next few days, and within two weeks "he was up and walking about." Nichols was given calomel and jalap to open his bowels and six leeches were applied to the testicles. In two weeks, Beaumont considered him healthy enough to be discharged.

It was Beaumont's great successes in dangerous and exacting cases like this one that gave him his reputation at the General Hospital. He was now second only to Widmer in surgical abilities and the two often worked together on difficult patients. Charles K. Clarke (1857-1924) has recorded Dr. Arthur Jukes Johnson's famous tale of the day Beaumont and Widmer operated on a native Canadian.[91]

"One day," Johnson said, "an Indian was brought in to have a cataract removed from his eye. The Indian could speak no English but had an interpreter with him. Dr. Beaumont, one of the most patient and painstaking of men, tried for over an hour to get the Indian to keep still while he attempted to cut out the cataract, but it was of no use; every time the knife approached the eye the man would either turn his head, or close his eyes, or do something else which made it impossible for the doctor to operate." At each interruption, Beaumont would "remove his spectacles, take his handkerchief out, and wipe the right glass of it [sic] — he had only one eye himself, although no one would ever suspect it."

Beaumont was eventually saved by the timely arrival of Widmer, dressed in what Johnson called his usual attire: riding breeches, top boots and riding crop.

"What's this you have here, Beaumont?" he asked of the exasperated surgeon.

Beaumont explained his difficulty and Widmer turned to the interpreter.

"Do you speak English?" he asked.

"Yes, sir," came the reply.

"Well," Widmer responded, "you can just tell this man that if he does not keep his head still and his eyes open he will go to the happy hunting ground so damned blind that he will never be able to find his way about."

As Johnson recalls, after Widmer had spoken, "the operation went on without the patient moving a muscle" and Beaumont successfully cut out the cataract.

Of more than passing interest is the reference to Beaumont's having only one eye. He started having problems with his sight in the mid-1850s and by 1865 was totally blind in his left eye. The sight in his right eye was also to fail him a few years later. Still, at the time of this story in 1858 his eyesight was good enough to handle complicated operations that put most of the other doctors in the hospital to shame.

For Widmer, however, his operating days were already over. When not keeping patients in line with savvy comments, he kept himself busy with administrative duties and teaching, but in truth he was declining fast, and it was only a short time later that he passed away. The date was 3 May 1858. He was 77 years old.

Beaumont must have been hard hit by his friend's death. Widmer had always been willing to use his considerable influence to help advance Beaumont's career and in general for more than 15 years had been a constant companion, valued colleague and helpful mentor.

With Widmer gone, the Trustees looked to a successor. It was no surprise when, in June 1858, they selected Beaumont as the hospital's consulting surgeon and *de facto* leader. Thus Beaumont now became the most influential surgeon at Toronto General Hospital in addition to being a significant force on the Medical Board and at the university. As well, he continued to fulfil an important role in the local Medico-Chirurgical and Ethical Society. (As vice-president with Hodder of this society, he endeavoured — albeit unsuccessfully — to promote "a code of ethics for the guidance of the profession" in the Toronto area.)

* * * *

A year after Widmer's death, Beaumont treated the unusual head injury described in the Prologue at the beginning of this book. The injury occurred when a portion of a flying wooden rocket buried itself in the skull of 45-year-old James Watkins. In a state of shock, he walked about 30 yards (27 metres) to the Shakespeare Tavern and friends immediately sent for a doctor.[92]

About fifteen minutes later, Beaumont arrived. The only sign of injury was the rocket shaft protruding out of the left eye-socket. Beaumont laid Watkins on the floor and propped up his head and shoulders. Surrounded by curious onlookers, he tried to take out the projectile with a pair of "tolerably strong forceps," but found it would not budge.

Beaumont sent for a pair of pliers. "Knowing that the shaft of a rocket is not round, like an arrow, but square, I was aware of the small extent to which it could be rotated on its axis," he wrote. "Still I found, on trying to do so, that a slight degree of movement on its axis was not impossible, and by turning it several times a few degrees alternately to the right and to the left I at last loosened it, and slowly drew out inch after inch of the shaft, with no small astonishment as the last two or three inches [five to seven centimetres] showed themselves." There was good reason for amazement. When it was fully withdrawn, the wooden shaft proved to be 15 centimetres long.

Before Beaumont moved the shaft there had been almost no bleeding, but that changed as soon as he pulled it out. "Its extraction was instantly followed by a profuse gush of blood — a stream almost as large as the extracted shaft."

Beaumont quickly covered the wound and applied ice water. His prompt action worked and within ten minutes the bleeding had stopped. Beaumont heaved a sigh of relief.

Despite the loss of blood, Watkins "did not even faint, and in less than 15 minutes, without any help, [he] got up from off the floor, and walked, saying that he felt quite able to do so. I directed his friends to keep him perfectly motionless, to apply unremittingly iced water to his head and to carry him gently to the hospital. I also prescribed small and repeated doses of calomel and jalap."

Watkins's friends paid no attention to Beaumont. Instead, they took him back to his boarding house on Queen Street and placed him under the care of the Irish doctor Charles William Buchanan. Canniff tells us that Buchanan was "one of the best known and highly respected medical men in the city."[93] He had been educated at Dublin, London and Glasgow and had been practising in Toronto since 1842 out of his house at 51 Adelaide Street West. He lived, therefore, quite close to Watkins and could watch him closely during his recovery.

A month later Beaumont and Watkins met again. Beaumont "found him in good health, strong, and perfectly well except for the total loss of sight of the left eye." Watkins said he had been up and walking within three days of the accident and that the wound had healed "very rapidly."

Beaumont could hardly believe Watkins' good fortune. He composed a clinical lecture based on the case and sent the text to the *Lancet*, which published it on 14 June 1862. Beaumont told his readers that "the patient's escape from death renders the case one of the most remarkable in the annals of surgery." The *Lancet* agreed, and so did London's Royal College of Surgeons, which eventually acquired the offending rocket-shaft for its museum.

In the spring of 1862 Beaumont saw Watkins again and found he had "remained nearly the same in every respect, his health and strength good, but his memory decidedly impaired."

Overall, the case caused much comment and debate in professional circles, both in Canada and Europe. Even a decade later it was still being described with amazement in the medical journals.

* * * *

Beaumont's reputation continued to soar. By the early 1860s he was the city's premier physician, and as such was given the most demanding and dangerous medical cases at the hospital. But dramatic lifesaving operations on critically wounded patients were the exception. He spent far more time dealing with routine cases, and as a result was constantly working on new ways to handle familiar tasks.

By 1860, operations for cataracts had ceased to challenge him as in the old days. Yet he continued to refine his instrumental skills. He developed a new sliding iris forceps to handle the difficult problem of removing portions of the iris without tearing the cornea on the way out. He came up with this particular innovation after using the fixed and sliding blade iris forceps of the German ophthalmologists Langenbeck and Graefe. Beaumont found the hook in the sliding blade of Langenbeck's forceps "objectionable" and inconvenient, while Graefe's forceps placed the sliding blade in a very awkward position, forcing the surgeon to use his thumb to move it back and forth, thus giving rise "to a want of precision in seizing the exact part of the iris" that Beaumont wanted.

So he tinkered with both instruments and developed a "final version" free of these encumbrances. Essentially he created an iris forceps with a hook that could be hidden when it was not needed, which made the instrument far easier to use. In his words, "the point of the hook is not only more concealed, but its concavity is quite filled by the end of the sliding blade, ie, when the blades are closed, so that the whole of the piece of the iris taken up by the hook is securely held. The form of the hook is also different, being less curved and rather larger [than those of its predecessors]."

The Beaumont forceps looked like a pen and was held in roughly the same manner, with the index finger being used to retract the blade. His description of its use is helpful: "In using the instrument it should be held as seen in the sketch, pressed by the thumb against the point of the middle finger, and against the proximal phalanx of the index...the point of the index finger being quite free to move without in the least displacing the point of the hook. It may be passed through a small puncture of the cornea, either with the blades closed or with the sliding blade drawn back about one tenth of an inch [25 millimetres], the point of the hook being exposed, and ready to take up the exact part of the iris intended to be seized. The hook should be passed through the plane of the iris very obliquely, so as to avoid wounding (in places where there is no cataract) the capsule of the lens; and then the point of the index finger (which has held back the sliding blade) being merely raised from the instrument, the sliding blade shoots forward, and its end jams up in the concavity of the hook, the piece of iris taken up by the latter. The extraction of a sufficient piece of iris through the wound in the cornea is easily effected, provided that the posterior surface of the iris be not unusually firmly adherent to the capsule of the lens."

Beaumont used his new instrument on a 50-year-old woman who was admitted to the Toronto General Hospital on 6 November 1860. He tells us she was in poor shape, with "the pupil of her right eye being almost obliterated, behind it a whitish opacity (cataract), and the cornea opaque at its lower and outer part. In the left eye was a soft cataract, its colour bluish-white." He operated twice on the left eye and restored its sight. In May, June and July of the following year he operated three times on the right eye, using the new iris forceps on each occasion. By the time Beaumont examined her again on 17 July 1861, "with a glass of four inches [10 centimetres] focus, she could readily tell the head of an ordinary pin from its point."

As a result of his continued successes in cases like these, Beaumont was elected a member of the Paris-based Société Universelle d'Ophthalmologie in 1861.

He continued to refine his iris forceps over the next few years and used them on several cataract patients, though not always with success.

In March and April, 1863, he used the device on a totally blind 40-year-old male patient at the Toronto General Hospital. Beaumont operated twice on the right eye, which had a large cataract and an "almost obliterated pupil," and formed an artificial pupil. But the patient did not get his sight back and by the end of April Beaumont still had not operated on the cataract itself.

His tardiness may have been due to the large number of cases he had to handle. On 14 March 1863 another a totally blind cataract case came into the hospital, a 27-year-old man with chronic iritis in the right eye, an adherent and contracted pupil and a large white cataract. Beaumont operated on March 27, puncturing the cornea, breaking the cataract and trying to tear off the adhesions on the pupil. He was unsuccessful, finding them "too firm to yield to moderate force." Not daring to pull any harder to break down the adhesions, he "passed into the anterior chamber the iris forceps described, seized the iris close to the temporal side of the pupil, and tore away a strip of it, leaving an artificial pupil on the outer and lower side of the iris." His patient felt some pain during the night, but none after that and the eye did not get infected. Shortly after, Beaumont removed the broken cataract fragments.

Overall, however, Beaumont was impressed enough with the success of his new iris forceps to submit a description of the device to the Royal Medical and Chirurgical Society of London, where it was read at the June meeting and subsequently published in the *Medico-Chirurgical Transactions* in 1863. Although strictly speaking not a new instrument so much as a modification of a combination of Beaumont's own design and the designs of others, a brief notice also appeared in the *Lancet*, and the Royal College of Surgeons in London was sufficiently impressed to put a copy of the instrument in their museum.

Beaumont's ingenuity is also revealed in the materials used in the manufacture of his instruments. In mid-nineteenth century Canada, medical-instrument makers were few and far between and improvisation was common. The iris forceps had a handle made from a simple silver tube and a piece of cedar. More significantly, "the fixed blade, the hook, is made of a moderate- sized sewing needle, the point of which is easily curved after softening it a very little."

* * * *

Although Beaumont's inventions generally won him great acclaim, not all his innovations were successful. On 13 January 1863, for example, Richard Humphreys died in the Toronto General Hospital from an overdose of chloroform while under the care of Beaumont and Hodder.[94]

Chloroform, introduced in 1847 in Edinburgh as an anaesthetic in obstetrics by Simpson, had quickly superseded ether. Beaumont first used it around 1847-1848 and was justifiably proud of his success with it. Although scarcely a month went by when he did not read about a death due to chloroform overdose in the hospitals of England or France, he had not once had a mishap with it. By 1863, physicians at the Toronto General Hospital had successfully used chloroform nearly 2000 times.

Humphreys entered the hospital around January 7, suffering from a tumour. Beaumont, Hodder, Bovell and King consulted with Michael Lawlor and J. Gardiner, two newer hospital staff doctors, and the six physicians decided to operate to remove the tumour. Beaumont and Hodder would perform the surgery while Bovell and Gardiner administered chloroform. King and Lawlor would be "at hand to lend any assistance that might be necessary."

Before Humphreys consented to the use of a general anaesthetic, he told his wife and fellow patient Edward Fawcett that "he would go to the operating table prepared to die, as all persons should do in his opinion who were operated under the influence of chloroform." It was a sadly prophetic statement. As soon as Beaumont and Hodder started operating, "the pulse of the patient ceased acting, the face assumed a pallid hue, and respiration ceased."

A few days later, Beaumont described in more detail what happened: "After Dr. Hodder commenced the operation, Dr. Bovell made an exclamation to the effect that the patient's face was in danger from chloroform.

I was assisting Dr. Hodder at the operation, and left my post for a moment to examine the patient, which had a death-like pallor. The pupils of both eyes were greatly dilated. I immediately gave a pair of hooked forceps, I believe, to Dr. Bovell, to draw forward the tongue, in order to prevent the closing of the passage into the windpipe. Electricity was immediately employed and Dr. Bovell and myself produced artificial respiration by compressing the walls of the chest, and obtaining that [by] allowing its [the chest's] dilatation. In a very short time there seemed a slight change — toward resuscitation — indicated by contraction of the pupils, and it was thought by some of the medical men present that there was some slight return of respiration, the veins of the neck were turgid and one was opened by Dr. Gardener. Everything proved unavailing."

The medical team tried every means known at the time to revive Humphreys: chemical stimulants, artificial respiration, electrical stimulation over the phrenic nerve in the neck to start breathing again. In opening the jugular vein, Gardiner had hoped "to relieve the pressure on the brain," which was thought to be a factor in the patient's collapse. But only two ounces of blood were collected, because by that time the patient was dead.

A post mortem revealed that Humphreys had died from "cerebral apoplexy." In other words, his brain had suffered a stroke as a result of the chloroform. Because this complication had never been reported before, an inquest was called and Beaumont, Hodder and the others present at the operation were called by coroner William Hallowell to give evidence. Both Fawcett and Mrs. Humphreys testified that the dead man had been a "hale, strong, hearty man". There was no apparent reason for his death, but there it was. In the opinion of the doctors involved, the death was an unpredictable accident.

Aikins and Wright, who had fought so bitterly with Beaumont, now rallied to his defence with a statement that "from the evidence [they had heard], and the report of the postmortem operation, that everything had been done that was possible under the circumstances; and that no blame was attached to anyone, and that the medical gentlemen were justified in using the chloroform from the appearances of the patient, notwithstanding the unfavourable result." They had forgiven the Trustees for their 1855 dismissal and had forgotten the diaries of Beaumont's incompetence. They were willing to work together peacefully once more.

The jury concluded that "Richard Humphreys came to his death from apoplexy, induced by chloroform, which we believe, from the evidence, was properly administered, and that the best means were adopted for his resuscitation."

Despite the verdict, the *Daily Globe* continued to criticize the medical profession after the inquest. It argued that local doctors, in a bid to attract customers, gave chloroform too freely to timid patients who feared pain above all else. The editors wrote that Humphreys' death "presents a very startling picture, which ought, it seems to us, afford a practical lesson of great importance. Humphreys was a strong and healthy man, in the prime of life, who found it needful to submit to an operation for a very common and not dangerous disease. He came to Toronto for the benefit of the best medical aid, he was laid upon the operating table, surrounded by men who are at the head of their profession in Canada, and in a few minutes he was a corpse."[95]

What, the *Globe* asked, was the moral to be drawn from this sad tale? Simply this: "Nobody likes to suffer pain; everyone escapes it who can; and there is no doubt the present general use of chloroform is the work of the patient and not of the physician. But it is the duty of a surgeon to refuse to administer it."

Doctors paid scant heed to the advice. Chloroform was here to stay and one fatality in 16 years, while it might make patients more apprehensive, would not lead to its disuse.

* * * *

Beaumont's anguish over the loss of a patient was mitigated by the marriage, on 17 October 1863 of his daughter Charlotte to Toronto businessman Edgar John Jarvis (1835-1907) in St. James' Cathedral.[96] The son of Frederick Starr Jarvis (1786-1852) and Susan Isabella Jarvis (formerly Merigold), the groom was a real estate agent operating out of the Whittemore buildings in Toronto.

It was almost literally marriage to the boy next door. The Beaumonts lived at 118 Wellington Street; Jarvis lived at 248 Wellington Street. Edgar and Charlotte had a son, Edgar Beaumont Jarvis, on 7 July 1864. At 61, William had become a grandfather. With Beaumont acting as one of the sponsors, Edgar was baptized by the Reverend Grasset in St. James' Cathedral on September 25. On 4 September 1865, Edgar and Charlotte had a second son, Paul Jarvis.

A year after their wedding, the couple moved, first to 218 Victoria Street, then, in 1866, to "Glenhurst, Yorkville," a house they had built in what is now the plush downtown Toronto residential area of Rosedale. At that time it was very much a suburb and was still undeveloped. Charlotte gave it the name "Rosedale" in 1866, helping Edgar to develop it. They lived at Glenhurst for 16 years until they built "Sylvan Tower" in 1880. Later they also built "Deancroft" and "Craigleigh," prominent local landmarks all.

Edgar continued to sell real estate until his death from paralysis on 15 January 1907. Charlotte fell victim at the age of 89 to cancer of the gall bladder.[97]

* * * *

Beaumont continued to teach through the 1860s while he also maintained his office practice at home and his post as Consulting Surgeon at the Toronto General Hospital. But, like Widmer before him, old age was creeping up on him.

Problems with his vision continued to plague him. He finally lost the sight in his left eye in 1865, and by 1871 the inflammation that had caused the condition had spread to his right eye. Two years later he was completely blind. But before that was to happen there was one more opportunity to come his way: the chance to fulfil a lifelong dream, and he was not about to throw it away.

— Chapter 11 —

Army Surgeon at Last

Beaumont's health and surgical skills gradually declined in the 1860s and he began to pass operations over to his younger, steadier colleagues. He continued to assist, however, routinely working with his old friend Hodder, his former student William Canniff and his colleague John Lizars, an Edinburgh trained doctor who had been practising in Ontario since 1856.

On one occasion, after successfully removing a tumour "with Professor Bethune" from a man's upper jaw, Lizars was surprised to learn in conversation with Beaumont on this type of operation that Beaumont himself had carried out a similar procedure several years earlier, making "...a curved incision from the angle of the mouth towards the ear...ending his incision at the mastoid process."

Even his long-time rival Aikins enjoyed Beaumont's assistance in the operating theatre, the two being friends once again, and Beaumont no longer finding the younger man "too inexperienced" to assist. At one point, Aikins described, for example, his efforts to remove a large tumour from the eye socket of an eight-year-old boy. With Beaumont's help, he was able to "scoop out the whole cavity" and remove a tumour the size of a man's fist. They concluded that while they had saved the patient, his long term chances were not good. "Although the boy is relieved of an offensive mass," Aikins wrote, "it is altogether likely that it will return in all virulence and ultimately secure its victim."

Also in the 1860s, Beaumont finally got the opportunity to fulfil the ambition to be an army doctor that he had cherished for over 30 years. His chance came in the summer of 1866 when the Fenian Raids brought Canada and the United States to the brink of war.

The Fenian Brotherhood was a group of Irish Americans with a complex history. Founded by Irish nationalists John O'Mahoney and James Stephens in New York City in 1857 and 1858, their original intention was to gain Ireland's independence from the British Empire. The name was derived from Fianna, the legendary defenders of Ireland during ancient times. At first the brotherhood developed slowly, but the movement gained great impetus during the American Civil War (1861-1865), when many Irish received military training while fighting for the Union Army. By 1865 the Fenians had split into two groups, one under O'Mahoney, raising money for an Irish uprising, the other under Colonel William Roberts and General Sweeney, preparing for an attack on Canada. The idea was that Britain would rush to the defence of Canada and become embroiled in a long-drawn war with the United States. When that happened, it was thought, Irish independence would be easily won.

In April 1866, O'Mahoney's group organized a gathering of forces on the New Brunswick border and briefly violated the British neutral territory of the island of Campobello. But British, colonial and American military forces quickly repulsed them and this phony "invasion" fizzled out. During May, however, hundreds of Fenians massed on the American-Canadian border from Detroit to St. Albans, Vermont. Fourteen thousand Canadian volunteer troops were called up on May 31 to prepare for the real Fenian invasion of Ontario.

They did not have long to wait. That evening, 800 Fenians under former Union Army officer John O'Neill invaded the Niagara peninsula and camped near Fort Erie until the evening of June 1. On the same day, 1240 Canadian volunteers were sent to Port Colborne, Ontario, and an additional 600 British troops arrived at Chippawa that night. They were heavily reinforced the next morning. The Port Colborne volunteer force under Colonel Alfred Booker set out to join up with the British troops — and met the Fenians near the village of Ridgeway. The volunteers retreated ignominiously back to Port Colborne, having lost ten men killed and 38 wounded. The Fenians retired to Fort Erie themselves, where they quickly dispatched a small Canadian force sent there by Colonel John Stoughton Dennis of Toronto. To avoid fighting the better-trained regulars, they then returned to the United States. The British refused to pursue them beyond the border and instead left it to the American government to step in and punish them. The invasion was a resounding failure, both politically and militarily: Britain and America had demonstrated that they were not willing to go to war over the Fenian cause after all.

The incident had given rise to some tense moments, however, and there had been a battle with men killed and wounded. Beaumont, ever loyal to the crown, was quick to offer his medical services, as were Dr. Ryall of Hamilton and William Canniff, then in Belleville. Their offer accepted, Beaumont and Ryall were placed in charge of a military hospital at Port Colborne on June 2, and Canniff arrived the next day.

Canniff describes the scene: "Our train reached Port Colborne about four in the afternoon. The place was thronged with the military and civilians. Already an hospital had been established here under the care of Surgeon Ryall of the 13th Batallion, and everything was being done that could possibly be done in the way of nursing, comforts, &c. Dr. Beaumont, of Toronto, was in constant attendance in consultation with Dr. Ryall. There were nearly 20 then in hospital. I did not examine many of the wounded. Indeed there seemed a serious danger that the crowd of medical men who had arrived, would prove to be deleterious to the wounded who so badly needed repose."[98]

A Dr. Elliott from Fort Erie also attended for a short while. The hospital now had four doctors for 20 patients. Canniff didn't stay very long, however. Instead, Ryall sent him to the front the next morning to take care of the wounded there while he and Beaumont continued to treat the patients at the hospital. A few more were added as the days passed, mostly Canadians, but also a couple of Fenians as well: one wounded in the scalp, the other in the groin.

Beaumont enjoyed his short stint as army surgeon, but the wounded were soon attended to and in mid June he returned to Toronto. He resumed his teaching duties at the hospital and his private practice.

Sadly, he had scarcely returned home before he lost his wife, Mary Catherine, at the age of 44. She had been ill for a considerable time, but finally, in 1866, consumption claimed her. Beaumont turned to his children and his ever-increasing family of grandchildren to ease the pain of his bereavement. He also still had many medical students to keep him company.

One of his most famous students was Sir William Osler (1849-1919) who, as Professor of Medicine, was to dominate the medical schools at Montreal's McGill University from 1874 to 1884, the University of Pennsylvania between 1884 and 1889, Johns Hopkins from 1889 to 1905 and Oxford from 1905 to his death. He is considered by some to have been "perhaps the most influential physician since Hippocrates."[99]

Osler spent only a few years in Toronto (he entered Trinity College in 1866 and left for McGill in 1870), but his formative schooling under Reverend William Johnson and Hodder and Bovell left an impression on him. Osler also had the opportunity to study under Beaumont from 1866 onwards and was clearly impressed with his master's abilities. In his 1904 *Aequanimitas* book of essays for medical students, Osler remarks that "in William R. Beaumont and Edward Mulberry Hodder, we had before us the highest type of the cultivated English surgeon." He added that "medicine is seen at its best in men whose faculties have had the highest and most harmonious culture...Beaumont, Bovell and Hodder in Toronto...these and men like unto them have been the leaven which has raised our profession above the dead level of a business."

Osler had good reason to be impressed with Beaumont, Bovell and Hodder, for at the time the three were involved in the carrying out of sophisticated operations for the removal of tumours and cysts from the ovaries.

One of their patients was a 32-year-old woman who required two operations for the removal of bilateral ovarian tumours. Hodder reported the case in the *Canada Lancet* in 1872, with acknowledgement to Beaumont.

By this time, Beaumont was doing more than giving younger doctors like Hodder the benefit of his experience. He was also instructing medical students at the very institution he had struggled against for years — the rival Toronto School of Medicine.

Beaumont had given up his professorship when the University of Toronto's Medical School was abolished by the Hincks Act in 1853. The Trinity College Medical School was shut down three years later as a result of squabbles over finances and religious tests. That left the Toronto School of Medicine as the dominant force in medical education. It had changed over the years, starting with incorporation in 1851. In 1854 it had joined with Victoria University, then at Cobourg, to become the university's Toronto campus medical department.

In 1856, several of the staff of the Toronto School of Medicine, among them Workman, Aikins and Wright, left Rolph and set up a new Toronto School of Medicine, leaving Rolph at Victoria to teach all the classes himself. Fortunately for him, he was soon joined by Geikie, Reid and others, but at first it was rough going. Now there were once again two medical schools in the city: the Rolph-dominated Victoria University Medical Department, and the new Toronto School of Medicine under president Aikins.

This situation remained unchanged until 1867 when, with Strachan's death in November of that year, one of the main obstacles to the lifting of religious tests at Trinity University was removed. In December 1867, Hodder and others began to revive the Trinity Medical School. In November 1870 Bovell, Hodder, Bethune, Hallowell and Cyrenius B. Hall were appointed to the Board of Medical Examiners at Trinity College.

Theological disputes had been resolved in a bizarre compromise whereby the religious declaration stayed on the University's books, but students were given the option of a dispensation. In practice, this meant that the religious requirement was dropped from the school. Classes started in October.

Thus the situation had changed drastically from what it had been when Beaumont was a university professor. Since his friends Hodder, Bovell, Richardson and others were already at the new Toronto School of Medicine, it is not hard to see why Beaumont eventually agreed to join that school. He began lecturing there in its 27th session, which ran from 1 October 1869, to 1 April 1870. Classes were held in the Medical School Building (Moss Hall) on the university campus, which the Toronto School of Medicine leased from the University of Toronto.

Aikins and the other faculty were delighted to have Beaumont on staff and wasted no time advertising his arrival to prospective medical students. "Since last session the lecturing staff has been strengthened," the *Annual Announcement of the School* reported in 1869, "by...Dr. Beaumont — for many years Professor of Surgery and Clinical Surgery in the University of King's College, Toronto — as lecturer on Diseases of the Eye, Vesical diseases, strictures, etc. The extended research and ripened experience of this master in Surgery cannot fail to enrich the minds of his pupils."

* * * *

Although he was lecturing again, Beaumont still had time to do a little surgical research of his own at the Toronto General Hospital. In September, 1870, he published an article on "Cases of Stone in the Bladder — Lithotrity [the crushing of a stone]" in the *Canada Lancet*,[100] based upon his clinical work at the Toronto Hospital over the previous two years.

The first operation described in this paper was for "a calculus [small stone] lodged in the urethra, near the neck of the bladder, which several times caused total retention of urine, which was relieved almost daily for about a week by Dr. Hampton," resident surgeon at the Toronto General Hospital, who was Gardiner's nephew. Beaumont crushed the stone by using an "old fenestrated form" of lithotrite, or crushing instrument. "He walked home immediately afterwards," Beaumont later wrote of his patient, "passed the fragments the next day, and remained well a long while afterwards when I last heard of him."

Beaumont had a more difficult time with his next patient, a "William T." who had been suffering from "severe symptoms of stone for about two years or rather more." Beaumont had to operate 15 times over seven months, using his largest lithotrite to crush over a hundred fragments of stone. After the second operation, the patient was in so much pain that Beaumont had to put him to sleep with chloroform. "A most enormous quantity was used," he admitted, "usually four, or five, or six ounces, before he became insensible." After the last operation Beaumont concluded that it was "a most troublesome case," but his patient was finally free from symptoms.

By the time of his next case, on 8 February 1870, he had acquired a new "flat-bladed lithotrite, recommended by Sir Henry Thompson" — an English specialist in urogenital tract surgery who had published several books, including the *Stricture of the Urethra* (1854), and *Practical Lithotomy and Lithotrity* (1863).

Beaumont notes: "It is made by Weiss, of London, and seems as perfect as a lithotrite can be; the sliding movement being instantly changed to the screw movement, and vice versa, the screw to the sliding movement." Beaumont the inventor conceded the importance of other doctors' tools when he needed them. The instrument was used on a 35-year-old "Thomas G." from Lucan, Ontario. Five sessions were required to crush the stone and all the fragments without complication and with complete relief of pain.

"Considering the size of the stone," Beaumont wrote, "its long continuance in the bladder, and its hardness, this was one of the most satisfactory cases of lithotrity one could have."

Beaumont was by now the expert in this field and could expect much better success than his colleagues. (One of Canniff's patients, for example, with a relatively minor single stone went into shock from haemorrhage and died soon after the operation.)

* * * *

Beaumont was active in efforts to improve medicine in Ontario by ridding it of "quack doctors." He was particularly hostile to two groups of alternative medical practitioners: the homeopaths and eclectics.

Homeopathy was advocated by Samuel Hahneman (1755-1843) at the beginning of the century. It was based on the principle that small doses of drugs cure diseases having the same symptoms produced by large doses of the same drugs in normal people. The eclectics took their inspiration from Samuel Thomson (d.1843), who argued that natural herbs and plants were all that was required to cure disease. Although both groups were in decline, they had been put on the same footing with orthodox medical doctors by the Ontario Medical Act of 1869.

On 8 March 1871, Beaumont chaired a meeting of about 30 Toronto doctors at the Mechanics' Institute. The group called for a repeal of the Act and reiterated that the medical profession should always be consulted by the government before any such legislation is passed into law. No such consultation had taken place. The members, agreeing with Beaumont's long- held opinion, carried his suggestions to the provincial government, but the Act was not amended until after Beaumont's death.

* * * *

Beaumont continued to teach at the Toronto School of Medicine until the end of term on 1 April 1871. Meanwhile, the revived School of Medicine at Trinity College was preparing to open. In March, the Trinity Corporation had hired Hodder, Bethune, Hallowell, Geikie and Rolph school graduate John Fulton as professors. Lectures were to begin on October 2 and to continue for six months. Beaumont could not resist an offer to join all his friends at Trinity. He was lured from the Toronto School of Medicine 8 March 1871, when he was elected Emeritus Professor of the Principles and Practice of Surgery at Trinity University. He worked at Trinity giving lectures and advice for the next four years until his death.

Already in the late 1860s, however, it was clear that Beaumont's time was running out. Although he was steadily reducing his clinical practice as a result of his ever-worsening eyesight, it was becoming increasingly obvious that full retirement would soon be necessary. About this time his son Herbert moved away from home and settled at 30 D'Arcy Street. Beaumont himself decided to move up to Yorkville to be closer to his daughter and did so just in time to welcome another grandson, Herbert Cherriman Jarvis, into the world on 17 October, 1871. It was the last grandchild he would see.

On 6 April 1872, Beaumont wrote his last will and testament. Half of his life insurance policy, savings accounts and silver plate was to go to Charlotte and the rest of his estate, after funeral expenses and debts had been deducted, was to be given to his son. Edgar Jarvis and Herbert Beaumont were appointed executors.

In 1873 Beaumont lost his sight entirely and he finally retired to his home in Yorkville.

On 19 May 1874, Edgar and Charlotte gave him another grandson, Louis Raymond Jarvis.

Beaumont passed many of his declining days with his grandchildren at the Jarvis home in Glenhurst, Toronto, and it was there, on 12 October 1875, that he eventually succumbed to paralysis.[101]

His will was probated at $5461.27, which included the Wellington Street house ($2000) and his bank account ($400). The rest of the estate was made up of silver plate ($159), medical books ($138) and surgical instruments ($159). Since a finely crafted Beaumont ophthalmological instrument would fetch $6, the value of his personal surgical instruments was substantial at $159. The fate of the instruments is not known. The valuation might have been simply an estimate, but it could have been the proceeds from their sale. If so, it is likely that most of them were subsequently lost or destroyed.

Chapter 12

Did Beaumont Invent the Sewing Machine?

Beaumont's reputation today tends to rest more on his supposed contributions to the early history of the sewing machine than it does on his contributions to medical education, public and professional governance and his flair for surgical instrumentation. If, as so many historians of Canadian medicine have argued, Beaumont was indeed the inspiration behind the sewing machine, the claim would be something to shout about indeed. After all, mechanized sewing revolutionized many industries in the nineteenth century and contributed to the introduction of mechanization in the home.

"The impact of the sewing machine was felt throughout the world...In light engineering it created the great sewing-machine industries of the United States from the 1850s, and of Germany from the 1870s, supplying machines for both industrial and commercial use. As an article of commerce, 'the first consumer appliance' became the most widely advertised and distributed product of the modern world...The 'iron seamstress' occasioned perhaps the last machine-breaking riots; pre-eminently a labour-saving device, it effectively ended the traditional bondage of women to the needle."[102]

How did Beaumont come to be credited with this role?

Virtually all modern biographies of William Beaumont trace the story back to a single source: the obituary notice in the *Canada Lancet* of 1 November 1875 in which Beaumont is correctly described as having "invented and made for himself several surgical instruments, some of which are of great ingenuity and utility."

He is credited with an instrument "for passing sutures in deep-seated parts (as in the operation for cleft palate), which was examined and admired by Brunel, the great engineer, and was reputed by Tiemann, surgical instrument maker of New York, to have been the origin of the Singer Sewing Machine. An account of it was published in the *Medical Gazette*, Dec. 3, 1836, and in the *Lancet*, 17th March, 1866. With it a continuous chain of stitches can be sewed, though in the operations for which it was invented but one at a time was required."

Other obituary notices turned out to be very similar to the one in the *Canada Lancet*. The *British Medical Journal* a month and a half later said that Beaumont "invented, and himself made, several surgical instruments of great ingenuity and utility," and that the 1836 cleft-palate device "was examined and admired by Brunel, the great engineer, and was considered by Tiemann, the surgical instrument maker in New York, to have been the origin of the Singer Sewing Machine."[103] Much the same phrases occur in a *Canada Medical and Surgical Journal* obituary that appeared in 1876. There is no doubt that both accounts of Beaumont's life came from the same sources as the *Canada Lancet*'s.

The *Canada Medical and Surgical Journal* provided sources with its obituary. "The data for this notice," it said, "have been supplied by Dr. Temple and H. Beaumont, Esq., and we are indebted to Dr. Zimmermann of Toronto, for sending us the facts in time for this number of the Journal."

The "H. Beaumont" is clearly William's son Herbert. He provided the facts about Beaumont's personal life and family.

James Algernon Temple was a McGill graduate of 1865, who, after a period of postgraduate training in England, returned to Toronto to practise with Hodder and teach at Trinity College Medical School. He was thus closely connected to Beaumont's circle of friends and professional colleagues and probably gave the journals details of Beaumont's medical career.

Richard Zimmermann was a Toronto doctor who practised from his home at the corner of Church and Richmond Streets. He was also on the staff of the Hospital for Sick Children at 31 Avenue Street and the Toronto Dispensary at 99 Adelaide Street West.

The Brunel mentioned in the obituaries could be either Sir Marc Isambard Brunel (1769- 1849), or his son Isambard Kingdom Brunel (1806-1859). Both were famous English inventors and engineers. The elder Brunel was a shipmaker and machinist best known for a tunnel he built under the River Thames in 1843. The younger Brunel was celebrated for bridges, railroads, canals and ships, his most famous being the Great Eastern steamship of 1859. Of the two, however, the father seems the most likely admirer. Among his lesser-known inventions were machines to make boots and knit stockings, so he would have likely been the more interested in Beaumont's surgical sewing tools.

George Tiemann (1795-1868) was one of the most important instrument salesmen in nineteenth century America. He also invented and manufactured devices of his own, and by the 1840s had become famous for his careful machining and innovative designs. The catalogues of Geo. Tiemann and Co., No. 67 Chatham Street, New York — well-studied during Beaumont's lifetime — contained several Tiemann inventions. The surgeon P. S. Townsend, for example, said that "the profession for many years owes much to Mr. Tiemann for the very perfect workmanship, not only of all the ordinary instruments employed in surgery, midwifery, &c., but also for the very great improvements he has made in some of them, and for those remarkable instruments of his own invention...which have justly given to this very scientific and intelligent artist an enviable reputation."

Both the *British Medical Journal* and the *Canada Medical and Surgical Journal* obituaries tell us a few important things the *Canada Lancet* does not. They point out that the story of Beaumont's discovering the principle of the sewing machine did not come solely from Brunel and Tiemann. The priority accorded to Beaumont was "shared by Sir James Paget and communicated by him to the late Dr. Fraser of Toronto...Our friend Mr. T.M. Stone, of the Royal College of Surgeons, who was a frequent correspondent of Dr. Beaumont, [also] claims this discovery for his friend, stating that long before the sewing machine was known, Dr. Beaumont had shown, and subsequently presented to him, the instrument."

Paget's contact with Beaumont dates back to their student days at St. Bartholomew's. He would have seen Beaumont's inventions almost as soon as they were put together and is known to have made extensive use of them. He believed in Beaumont's priority in sewing machine history. Paget also published a Beaumont obituary of his own in the *Proceedings of the Royal Medical and Chirurgical Society.*

What about Stone and Fraser? Little can be said about their role in the story, as their actual identities are uncertain.

There are two physicians named Stone in *Plarr's Lives of the Fellows of the Royal College of Surgeons*: Thomas Arthur Stone (1797-1864), an original Fellow and Harveian Orator, and Thomas Stone (1807-1877), a resident surgeon to Christ's Hospital. The former may be rejected on the basis of the middle name and the date of death. Thus the latter is most likely the man referred to in the obituaries.

The identity of Dr. Fraser is more obscure. There was a John Fraser practising medicine on Yonge Street in the 1870s who demonstrated anatomy at Trinity College, but he was still alive after Beaumont's death. Did the obituary make an error in mentioning the "late Dr. Fraser"? Or were there other Toronto doctors named Fraser at the time, as yet untraced?

There was very little recorded interest in Beaumont for 20 years after his death until Canniff published *The Medical Profession in Upper Canada, 1783-1850,* which included the biographies of almost 300 doctors, Beaumont among them. His account of Beaumont, complete with his version of the sewing machine story, was taken largely from the earlier medical journals. (Canniff did add a few notes about his own student days with Beaumont, however, and, more importantly, included the minutes of many of the early King's College Medical Department and Upper Canada Medical Board meetings, thus illustrating for the first time Beaumont's role in politics and administration.)

By the turn of the century, the beliefs and opinions of Tiemann and Paget had hardened into unshakeable convictions and a subtle change began to appear in the chronicles. Charles Clarke, in his 1913 *History of the Toronto General Hospital* (in addition to including some hitherto unpublished accounts of Beaumont's clinical work at the hospital) said "there is not the slightest doubt that it [Beaumont's invention] served as the model for the sewing machine." He added that a copy of the instrument had been stored at the Toronto Hospital for many years but had subsequently been lost. M. Charlton (1921) and Thurston Scott Welton (1935) stated flatly that the instrument "served as the model for the Singer Sewing Machine Company."

In England, however, D'Arcy Power's 1930 revision of *Plarr's Lives of the Fellows of the Royal College of Surgeons of England* finally gave actual details of the contents of the Beaumont medical papers cited by earlier biographers — and thus was among the first to cast suspicion on the tale. Power recalled that the 1866 Lancet obituary had indeed attributed Singer's inspiration for his sewing machine to Beaumont's instrument, but, Power pointed out, "the statement is not confirmed by the *Encyclopaedia Britannica*, Art. 'Sewing Machine.' (Vide E.A.J. Barker)."

With the seeds of doubt thus sown, subsequent authors returned to the more tentative nineteenth century notion that Beaumont's invention was believed only by *some* to have *possibly* been an inspiration for Singer.

These authors included George W. Spragge, whose important 1966 article clarifying the complex rivalry issues that had plagued medical schools in Toronto shed new light on Beaumont's role at Trinity College. Another was W.G. Cosbie, whose 1972 biography of Beaumont included a bibliography of Canadian sources, and whose 1975 history of Toronto General Hospital supplied additional details of Beaumont's clinical work. A third was Charles Godfrey, who included new details of Beaumont's life in Canada in his 1979 *Medicine for Ontario*.

Further doubts were cast in 1977 when Gary Bell published a short paper on the issue in the *Toronto Bulletin of the Academy of Medicine*. While working at the History of Medicine Museum of the Academy of Medicine in Toronto, Bell and his colleagues found a copy of the Beaumont invention that was said to have served as Singer's inspiration. The steel and brass cleft-palate instrument, complete with a small card associating it with the sewing machine, had been donated to the museum many years before by Dr. Newton Albert Powell.

Powell had studied medicine at Victoria University and Trinity College during the 1870s while Beaumont was still teaching in Toronto and had obtained his M.D. from the University of New York in 1875. After that, he had returned to Toronto to practise and had become head of the General Hospital's emergency department in 1908.

Intrigued with Powell's donation, Bell decided to thoroughly research the sewing machine story. He was not impressed with what he found. Apart from the fact that there was no evidence linking Beaumont and Singer in the first place, even if Singer had borrowed from Beaumont, all he might have found useful was a very small part of Beaumont's deep-suturing instrument.

"It is unnecessary to bolster additional support for Beaumont's reputation," he concluded, "by the introduction of a story of dubious historical merit."

Why was Bell so unequivocal in debunking the sewing machine tale? With a careful look at the articles cited in the obituaries, it is easy to see the answer. The *Canada Lancet* referred its readers to the 3 December 1836, *Medical Gazette* and the 17 March 1866 *Lancet* for supporting evidence. An examination of these two sources is revealing.

The *Medical Gazette* is in fact the *London Medical Gazette*, and the article referred to describes an 1836 instrument for closing recto-vaginal or vesico-vaginal fistulae that was discussed at length earlier. In this paper, Beaumont says the instrument was designed "for sewing together the edges of vesico-vaginal or recto-vaginal fistulae." It has an eye-pointed needle and can be used to form "a common or quilled suture." The instrument does not, however, contain the slightest hint of any potential for continuous mechanical action, or support for the material to be sewn, or a feeding mechanism to permit one stitch to follow the next, or tension controls to provide for even thread delivery, or any other feature commonly associated with a mechanical sewing device. In fact, the words "sewing machine" are never used.

Beaumont designed this instrument to allow for ease of recovery of the suture after each passage of the needle preparatory to rethreading the needle for its next passage. The instrument was intended to be used for making the "compound or quilled suture of the old surgeons" in deep wounds.

More to the point, however, is the fact that this instrument is not the 1837 deep-seated suturing device that was originally described by Power and credited by Paget as being the source of inspiration. There are two ways to explain this. Either the obituary writers never studied the 1836 article in depth and did not realize that there were two different instruments — one for fistula (1836) and one for cleft-palate (1837) — or they were indeed referring to the fistula instrument and later writers confused it with the other.

Still, it is strange that the authors were never aware of the potential confusion, for the 1866 *Lancet* announcement, barely a paragraph in length, explicitly and correctly states the main use for the 1836 instrument was for the repair of fistulae: "THE SEWING MACHINE — It may not be generally known, but the fact deserves to be recorded in THE LANCET, that the principle of passing and arresting the thread in Singer's Sewing Machine was taken from an instrument invented by a distinguished member of our profession, Mr. W. Rawlings [sic] Beaumont, of Toronto, an honorary fellow of the Royal College of Surgeons of England, who used the ingenious instrument for passing sutures in vesico- and recto-vaginal fistula. Singer took his idea from Mr. Beaumont's instrument exhibited in the shop of Freeman, a surgical instrument maker in New York."

Actually, this announcement raises more problems: the 1866 *Lancet* says that a surgical instrument maker named *Freeman* exhibited Beaumont's device, but in the *Canada Lancet* Singer is reputed by the well-known surgical instrument maker *Tiemann* to have taken his idea for the sewing machine from the device.

Are there two instrument makers, and if so, just who is Freeman? Perhaps the *Lancet* editor mistook "Freeman" for "Tiemann."

Bell says that Freeman was indeed a separate figure "contemporary with Tiemann." He goes on to say that "variations in the story indicate an element of unreliability and suggest that if there is confusion as to where the instrument was seen, there may be confusion as to whoever may have seen it, if indeed it was seen by anyone."

All these conflicting opinions demonstrate only one thing for sure: that it is impossible to be sure of anything! We do know that Beaumont invented a fistula instrument in 1836 and a deep-suturing device in 1837. We also know that these tools were widely used by nineteenth century surgeons, including Paget and Lawrence. Finally, we know that George Tiemann displayed and sold Beaumont's surgical instruments in his New York store.

Could Singer have seen the instruments on display? If he did see them, might he have drawn inspiration from them?

And what *of* Singer? When and where did he make his pioneering moves in sewing machine history? What does he say himself about the origins of his machine?

Among the most useful accounts in the well developed literature on the history of the sewing machine are the 1929 article by Frederick A. Lewton, "The Servant in the House: A Brief History of the Sewing Machine," and the Grace Rogers Cooper monograph of 1968, "The Invention of the Sewing Machine," both published by the Smithsonian Institution. It appears from these two articles that Singer in fact had very little to do with the invention of the original sewing machine. It was actually the work of many different inventors and by the time Singer came onto the scene a machine had already been on the market for many years.

The basic components of the sewing machine, it turns out, first appear in the latter half of the eighteenth century. Historians generally credit the German mechanic Charles F. Weisenthal with the 1755 development of the eye-pointed needle, and the English cabinet-maker Thomas Saint with the 1790 creation of a fabric support and vertical needle. John Duncan of Glasgow is usually considered to have made the first machine in 1804 that could create a chainstitch for embroidery with the simultaneous use of several hooked needles.

Thereafter, progress was rapid. Within three years the English machinists Edward and William Chapman patented the first machine that could sew with a needle that did not have its complete length passed through the fabric. Around 1810, German hosiery worker Balthasar Krems devised a machine that stitched circular peaked caps. It employed an eye-pointed needle used with a hook to make a chainstitch. By 1829 the French tailor Barthelemy Thimonnier had invented a machine that used a hooked needle to form a chainstitch on a fabric held horizontally. Finally, American mechanic Walter Hunt designed a sewing machine that created an interlocked or double-threaded stitch. However, he attached little significance to his creation and did not bother to patent it, later selling his machine to George Arrowsmith for a small sum.

Most historians give the American Elias Howe credit for inventing the first really practical sewing machine. Howe's machine, patented in 1846, used a curved eye-pointed needle carried by a vibrating arm with a spool supplying the thread. A thread carried by a moving shuttle locked loops of thread from the needle to create a lockstitch in a vertically mounted piece of fabric.

In October 1849, American inventor and tailor Sherburne C. Blodgett patented an entirely different principle using a circular, rotary shuttle rather than a reciprocating motion. It was this design that led to the first Isaac Merrit Singer sewing machine, which was built in September 1850 and patented in August 1851.

Singer dramatically improved the Blodgett machine by creating a horizontal platform to hold the cloth, a "yielding vertical presser foot" to keep the fabric in place as the needle was withdrawn and a vertically reciprocating needle driven by a rotary overhanging shaft. Virtually all these elements had already existed in varying combinations in earlier sewing machines, but Singer was the first to combine them into a practical, workable device that could be produced in large numbers and sold to the public. Thus, although he did not invent the sewing machine per se, he was responsible for turning it into a practical, mass-market product.

Singer was certainly successful in protecting his interests and aggressively marketing his new machine. He was sued for patent infringement by Howe in 1854 and lost the case, but the success of his machine took the sting out of the penalties imposed for patent infringement.

Singer subsequently patented 20 further improvements to his machine between 1851 and 1863 and hired a staff of more than 3000 to sell his product.

A rarity in 1851, by 1860 over 100 000 machines were being produced in the United States each year. Indeed, Singer's machine became so popular by the 1860s that many people equated the sewing machine's origin with him. Not surprisingly, popular science and technology writers impressed with his marketing success also commonly ascribed the invention to him.

Is it possible that among all the improvements constantly being made by Singer to his machine, some of them may have come from Beaumont's surgical instruments?

Bell says no. He argues that "the sewing machine is a complex object and the only significant feature for its design derived from Beaumont's instrument would be the eye-pointed needle."

Leaving aside the fact that the eye-pointed needle was invented by Weisenthal about 80 years before Beaumont started designing instruments, the eye-pointed needle appears in the Krems 1810 machine, as well as in the Hunt device of 1832-34 and the Howe machine of 1846. It is far more likely that Singer would have borrowed this feature from another sewing machine designer, for he was by his own admission working on improving their machines, not surgical instruments.

Is it possible, then, that Singer might have borrowed other ideas from Beaumont's instruments displayed or discussed in New York?

Singer, a native of Pittsdown, New York, first developed his machine between 1849 and 1851, 12 years or more after the publication of Beaumont's designs. He used the Boston machine shop of Orson C. Phelpes in Harvard Place, though he was often in New York City. (Indeed, when the machine was perfected in August 1850, Singer took the device to New York the very next day). However, there were many competing sewing machines in use by then, both in New York and Boston, and it seems more likely that Singer's ideas would have come from the Blodgett and Howe machines rather than from surgical tools.

Singer did in fact cite the Blodgett machine as one of the inspirations in his personal account of his invention. This fact was given as testimony during the 1854 patent infringement suit from Elias Howe. In answering the suit, Singer had to explain how he got the idea for the sewing machine independently of Howe. It would have been a strong argument in his defence had he claimed Beaumont as his source, but Beaumont's name was never mentioned — and there was no reference to surgical tools.

Singer put the process of discovery in this way in his defence against Howe: "I explained to them [Phelpes and machinist George Zieber] how the work was to be fed over the table and under the presser-foot, by a wheel, having short pins on its periphery, projecting through a slot in the table, so that the work would be automatically caught, fed and freed from the pins, in place of attaching and detaching the work to and from the baster plate by hand, as was necessary in the Blodgett machine."

Reflecting on these faults, Singer built an improved machine in 11 days, but it would not work. That night, Singer related, he and Zeiber "started for our hotel. On the way we sat down on a pile of boards, and Zieber mentioned that the loose loops of thread were on the upper side of the cloth. It flashed upon me that we had forgotten to adjust the tension on the needle thread. We went back, adjusted the tension, tried the machine, sewed five stitches perfectly and the thread snapped, but that was enough. At 3 o'clock the next day the machine was finished."

It is reasonable to conclude from statements like these that Singer developed his machine by seeing design flaws in the Blodgett instrument. Even allowing for the fact that Singer's story was given for self-serving ends, it seems likely that the principle of "passing and arresting the thread," which was never clearly defined in the *Lancet* piece, was a product of this 12-day period of design rather than the deliberate theft of Beaumont's ideas.

Consider the context of Singer's testimony. He was being sued for patent infringement to the tune of $25 000 by Howe, who had built and patented a working sewing machine in 1846, five years before Singer's. As Singer could hardly deny that Howe was the first to register his patent, his lawyer, Edward Clark, argued that Howe's patents were invalid because Hunt's obscure 1832 machine had been in operation long before.

Unfortunately for Singer, this argument did not succeed. Hunt was unable to produce a sample of his 1832 machine, and he had no patent on his design to offer as alternative evidence. The court upheld Howe's patent. In July 1854 Singer was forced to take out a licence from Howe and to pay him $15 000 in royalties for machines made before that date.

Singer would have been anxious to prove that Beaumont had anticipated them all. If he could have shown that the principles of the sewing machine had been in general use since Beaumont's 1836 and 1837 inventions, or that he had known about them when making his own machine, it would have saved him a lot of money, time and effort, for the law did not permit the patenting of a device that had already long been in the public domain.

Singer was searching hard for precedents when he gave his testimony, yet he failed to mention Beaumont. The only reasonable explanation is that he simply did not know Beaumont's instruments existed. And why should he? He was a machinist, not a surgeon.

Coupled to this is the curious omission of Beaumont's instruments from the catalogues of the day, particularly those published for George Tiemann and Company in New York. They show neither his fistula tool of 1836 nor his deep suturing instrument of 1837. Beaumont's opthalmology instruments were popular, but the early "sewing" devices do not appear to have been widely manufactured or advertised in the United States.

Why, then, did the 1866 *Lancet* make the claim for Beaumont's priority at all, particularly so long after the fact? Singer sewing machines were patented in 1851. Their origins were being debated by 1854, and the machines themselves were well known by 1860. Should not the arguments for priority have been presented at those times? How or why this unusual piece of "medical news" got into the *Lancet* in the first place is uncertain. It may be that Beaumont himself innocently sowed the seed.

In May 1863, Beaumont's paper on a "new iris forceps" appeared in the *Medico-Chirurgical Transactions*. Is it possible it accidentally set in motion a chain of events that led to the *Lancet* claim of 1866? In describing the forceps, Beaumont said he used "a moderate-sized sewing-needle, the point of which is easily curved by softening it a very little." Beaumont clearly used sewing tools in his practice whenever necessary and was not afraid to modify them when the occasion demanded.

Perhaps someone reading this 1863 article was led to compare the 1836 or 1837 instrument with the well-publicized Singer machine and,

1836 or 1837 instrument with the well-publicized Singer machine and, being unfamiliar with the long early history of the sewing machine, mistakenly informed the *Lancet* of Beaumont's priority. That would account for the wording of the 1866 piece. It would also explain why Beaumont rather than Howe or Hunt was credited with having inspired Singer.

Unfortunately there is no clue as to the identity of the source. It would have had to be someone conversant with Beaumont's work, yet unfamiliar with the history of the sewing machine. Stone, Fraser or Paget are candidates, but it could have been almost anyone.

The conclusion, then, must be that Singer did not copy Beaumont's work for any part of his invention, including the eye-pointed needle and the method of arresting the thread.

Could the sewing machine, on the other hand, have inspired Beaumont in designing his instruments?

Beaumont always designed his artifacts in response to practical surgical problems. He was quick to point out the improvements in his designs over the instruments that they replaced and he seldom described them without examples of their use on patients under his care.

Even so, it *is* possible that the eye-pointed needle of the 1836 and 1837 instruments came from the sewing machine tradition.

The Thomas Saint sewing machine had been patented in England as far back as 1790, but there were no contemporary references to its use and it was apparently little known. The same cannot be said of the Duncan and Chapman machines, however. The Glasgow Duncan sewing machine was patented in 1804 and its eye-pointed needle was used in embroidering machines for several years throughout Britain. The Chapman sewing machine, produced in London from 1807 onwards, also employed an eye-pointed needle. Beaumont could well have taken the idea for his eye-pointed suturing needles from either of them.

Chapter 13
Conclusion

Although Beaumont was a magnificent inventor of surgical instruments, he cannot be credited with the original concept of the sewing machine. Isaac Singer's sewing machine owed nothing to the surgical instruments of William Beaumont — neither the whole idea, nor any of its parts. Indeed, Singer himself had very little to do with the invention of the machine. He popularized it and made it a practical article of mass production. But the principles he supposedly borrowed from Beaumont were already long known by the time Beaumont embarked on his inventive career. The eye-pointed needle dated back to the previous century while the principle of passing and arresting the thread had also received practical application long before Singer's time. It was the integration of all the parts that made a working sewing machine possible, which had already been accomplished by inventors like the Chapmans, Krems, Thimonnier, Hunt and Howe. In fact, each of them (except Howe) developed their machines several years before Beaumont perfected his deep-suturing instrument. If there was any traffic in ideas, it is likely to have been in the opposite direction — from the sewing machine to Beaumont. It is even more probable that Beaumont derived some elements of his 1836 vaginal fistula instrument and his 1837 deep suturing instrument from sewing machines made years before.

If Beaumont didn't invent the sewing machine, why is he important to the history of Canadian medicine?

Beaumont was the first professor of surgery at the highly influential medical faculty of King's College, which later became the University of Toronto. This was one of the two earliest medical schools in Ontario (Rolph's School was the other) and was therefore crucial to the training of the next generation of Ontario doctors. Beaumont became the dean of the faculty.

Later in his life he taught at the Toronto School of Medicine and, in the 1870s, added to his achievements a professorship at Trinity University. In fact Beaumont worked for all the early medical schools of Toronto at one time or another and brought up a constellation of students that was to profoundly influence the course of medicine: William Osler, Uzziel Ogden, William Aikins, James Richardson, William Canniff and many others.

Beaumont's activity in medical administration is the least known aspect of his life. He was an energetic member of the Upper Canada Medical Board and was the leading figure in the upgrading of standards for the practice of medicine in Ontario. Moreover, his was a consistent voice promoting both medical incorporation and professionalization. He was a key player on the various governing boards of King's College and the University of Toronto. His roles in the upgrading of the Toronto General Hospital and the Insane Asylum are the best known of his administrative successes.

But it is his surgical techniques and instrumentation that will keep the memory of Beaumont alive. The claim that Beaumont was "the father of surgical instruments in Upper Canada" is no exaggeration, even without the Singer connection. Beaumont's devices contributed to the mechanization of medical practice in Canada, a trend that was the forerunner of technological development in all branches of medicine, particularly in surgical instrumentation.

Beaumont was among the first to use chloroform in Upper Canada and was experienced in the use of ether and nitrous oxide. During his years at the Toronto General Hospital he expanded the range of medical care that institution could offer by successfully demonstrating that difficult operations in ophthalmology, lithotomy, aneurysms and facial reconstruction were reasonable, not foolhardy undertakings.

Beaumont was prominent among the exemplars Osler encouraged his students to emulate. Osler was less concerned about achievement, however impressive, than a physician's attitude towards patients and the profession. He saw in Beaumont a commitment to patients and students from which he would not be deflected. It was not for his instruments or surgical techniques alone that Osler dubbed Beaumont "the highest type of cultivated English surgeon."

CONCISE LIST OF SOURCES

"A Medical Student," *Toronto Daily Colonist* (March 24, 1855).

"Correspondence: The University of Toronto and Medical Profession of Western Canada," *The British American Journal of Medical and Physical Science*, 6 (1850-1851), 42-44, 140-141, 189- 191, 285-286.

"Deaths," *Toronto Mail*, 4, #1108 (Wednesday, October 13, 1875), p. 1.

"Died," *Toronto Globe*, 32, #245, whole number 7979. (Wednesday, October 13, 1875), p. 2.

"Died," *Toronto Globe*, 32, #246, whole number 7980. (Thursday, October 14, 1875), p. 2.

"Important Medical Case: Inquiry into a Death from Chloroform," *The Daily Leader*, 10, #2979 (Thursday, January 15, 1863), 3.

"King's College, Toronto," *The British Journal of Medical and Physical Science*, 3 (1847-1848), 25.

"Licentiates of the Medical Board of Upper Canada," *The British American Journal of Medical and Physical Science*, 3 (1847-1848), 250.

"Medical Faculty," *Annual Announcement of the Medical Department, University of Trinity College, Session 1872-1873* (Toronto: Dudley and Burns, 1872), 2.

"Medical Faculty," *Annual Announcement of the Medical Department, University of Trinity College, Session 1873-1874* (Toronto: Dudley and Burns, 1873), 3.

"Medical Faculty," *Annual Announcement of the Medical Department, University of Trinity College, Session 1875-1876* (Toronto: Dudley and Burns, 1875), 2.

"Meeting of Medical Practitioners," *Upper Canada Journal of Medical, Surgical and Physical Sciences*, 2 (1852-3), 107-12.

"Meeting of the Medical Profession at Toronto," *Canada Lancet*, 3, #8 (April, 1871), 341-342.

"Minutes of the Proceedings of the Council of King's College at a meeting held on the 25th day of September, 1843," *King's College Council Minute Book, III* (Nov. 1842-Dec. 1848), 19-20, in Board of Governors, A70-0024, in

University of Toronto Archives, Toronto, Ontario.

"Mr. Beaumont on Fractures," *Medico-Chirurgical Review*, New Series, 16 (January 1, 1832), 247-51, p. 248.

"Mr. William Smith O'Brien in Toronto," *The Daily Globe*, 16, #107 (whole number 2832), (Thursday, May 5, 1859), 3.

"Obituary — W. R. Beaumont, F.R.C.S., England," *Canada Medical and Surgical Journal*, 4 (1876), 238-240.

"Obituary, William Rawlins Beaumont, M.D., F.R.C.S. Eng.," *British Medical Journal*, 2 (December 11, 1875), 749-750.

"Rosedale Pioneer is Taken by Death," *Toronto Globe* 88, #25 396 (Monday, May 22, 1931), p. 14.

"Royal Medical and Chirurgical Society, Tuesday, March 14, 1837," *London Medical Gazette*, 19 (Saturday, March 18, 1837), 938-939.

"The Act of Incorporation," *Upper Canada Journal of Medical, Surgical and Physical Sciences*, 2 (1852-1853), 167-174.

"The Death from Chloroform at the General Hospital," *The Daily Globe*, 20, #13 (Thursday, January 15, 1863), 3.

"The Late Dr. Beaumont," *Canada Lancet*, 8, #3 (November 1, 1875), 92-93.

"The Late Dr. Beaumont," *Toronto Mail*, 4, #1,109 (Thursday, October 14, 1875), p. 1.

"The Late Dr. Widmer," *The Daily Globe*, 12, #105, whole number 2518. (Tuesday, May 4, 1858), p. 3.

"The Medical Board," *Upper Canada Journal of Medical, Surgical and Physical Sciences*, 2 (1852-1853), 26-27; *Canada Medical Journal*, 1 (1852-1853), 191.

"The Rocket Accident on Wednesday Evening," *The Daily Globe*, 16, #108 (whole number 2833), (Friday, May 6, 1859), 3.

"The Sewing Machine" in "Medical News," *The Lancet* (March 17, 1866), 302.

"The Toronto General Hospital," *Upper Canada Journal of Medical, Surgical and Physical Sciences*, 2 (1852-1853), 280-288 [pagination irregular].

"The Use of Chloroform," *The Daily Globe*, 20, #14 (Friday, January 16, 1863), 3.

"Toronto General Hospital," *Upper Canada Journal of Medical, Surgical and Physical Science*, 3 (1853-1854), 29.

"Toronto Hospital," *The Semi-Weekly Leader*, 1, #73 (Tuesday, March 22, 1853), 2.

"Toronto University," *McKenzie's Weekly Message*, Toronto, Canada West, Thursday, March 3, 1853, #6, p. 1.

"Trinity College," *The Globe* (Toronto: Thursday, March 24, 1853), 143.

"Upper Canada Journal of Medical, Surgical and Physical Science," *The British American Journal of Medical and Physical Sciences*, 6 (1850-1851), 515-516.

Aikins, William Thomas, loose-leaf scrap book on medical education in Upper Canada at the Toronto Academy of Medicine.

Alphabetical Catalogue of the Library of the University of Toronto (Toronto: Henry Rowsell, 1857), 16.

American Armamentarium Chirurgicum: George Tiemann and Company's Surgical Instruments, 1889, reprinted and edited by Edmonson, James M., and Hambrecht, F. Terry (San Franciso: Norman Publishing, 1989).

Anderson, H.B., "The Medical Profession of Toronto," in Middleton, Jesse Edgar, *The Municipality of Toronto: A History* (Toronto: Dominion Publishing Company, 1923), 2, 609-628.

Annual Announcement of the Toronto School of Medicine, 27th Session, Oct. 1, 1869-April 1, 1870 (Toronto: Globe Printing Co., 1869), 4-5.

Annual Announcement of the Toronto School of Medicine, 28th Session, Oct. 1, 1870-April 1, 1871 (Toronto: Globe Printing Co., 1870), 4.

Annual Announcements, University of Trinity College Medical Reports, P78-0062 (.01-.04), University of Toronto Archives, Toronto, Ontario, Canada.

Armstrong, J., Rowsell's City of Toronto and County of York Directory for 1850-1 (Toronto: Henry Rowsell, 1850).

Beaumont, William (1785-1853), *Experiments and Observations on the Gastric Juice and the Physiology of Digestion* (Plattsburgh, New York: F. P. Allen, 1833; reprinted Cambridge: Harvard University Press, 1929).

Bebbington, Gillian, *London Street Names* (London: B.T. Batsford, 1972), 39, 215-216.

Bell, Gary, "Academy of Medicine — History of Medicine Museum; Registration Data Sheet," Catalogue Number X932.1.2, History of Medicine Museum, Academy of Medicine, Toronto, Ontario, Canada.

Bell, Gary, "William Rawlins Beaumont 1803-1875: An Inventor Surgeon," *Bulletin of the Academy of Medicine, Toronto*, 50, #3 (March, 1977), 49-51.

Bell, Kenneth, "Education, Secondary and University: Ryerson and Secondary Education" in Shortt, Adam and Doughty, Arthur G., ed., *Canada and its Provinces: A History of the Canadian People and their Institutions*, 18 (Toronto: T. and A. Constable, 1914), 372-373.

Bilson, Geoffrey, *A Darkened House: Cholera in Nineteenth Century Canada* (Toronto: University of Toronto Press, 1980).

Blondot, Nicholas, *Traité analytique de la digestion considérée particulièrement dans l'homee et dans les animaux* (Paris: Fortin, Masson et Cie., 1843).

Boase, Frederic, ed., "Beaumont, William Rawlins," in *Modern English Biography*, 1-6 (Truro: For the Author, 1892-1921; reprinted London: F. Cass, 1965).

Bonnycastle, Sir Richard, *The Canadas in 1841* (London: Henry Colburn, 1841), 1-2.

Boys, Henry, "University of King's College, Toronto: Hilary Term, 1844," *British Colonist*, 8, #2, (whole number 333), (Tuesday, January 9, 1844), page 3.

Britnell, W.E., ed., *County Marriage Registers of Ontario, Canada, 1858-1869*, 15 (Toronto City) (Agincourt: Generation Press, 1986), 8.

Brown's Toronto General Directory, 1856 (Toronto: W.R. Brown, 1856), 86, 106.

Brown's Toronto General Directory, 1861 (Toronto: W.C. Chewett and Co., 1861), 328.

Brown, George, *Brown's Toronto City and Home District Directory, 1846-7* (Toronto: George Brown, 1846), 30-31.

Brown, J.J., *Ideas in Exile* (Toronto: McLelland and Stewart, 1967).

Brunel, Isambard, *The Life of Isambard Kingdom Brunel, Civil Engineer: A Reprint with an Introduction by L. T. C. Rolt* (Rutherford, New Jersey: Fairleigh Dickinson University Press, 1972).

Bylebyl, Jerome J., "Harvey, William," in Gillespie, Charles Coulston, ed., *Dictionary of Scientific Biography* (New York: Charles Scribner's Sons, 1972) [hereafter D.S.B.], 6, 150-162.

Canniff, William, "Case of Epithelioma of the Tongue. Removal; Subsequent Return," *Canada Medical Journal*, 7(1870-1871), 405-407.

Canniff, William, "Experience among some of the Wounded who fell at the Battle of Limestone Ridge, June 2nd," *Canadian Medical Journal*, 2 (1865-1866), 529-534.

Canniff, William, *The Medical Profession in Upper Canada, 1783-1850* (Toronto: William Briggs, 1894; reprinted Toronto: Clarke, Irwin and Co., 1981), 243.

Catalogue Général des Livres Imprimés de la Bibliothèque Nationale: Auteurs, 9 (Paris: Imprimerie Nationale, 1902), 513.

Catalogue of Surgical Instruments Manufactured and Sold by Geo. Tiemann and Co. (New York: Geo. Tiemann and Co., 1872).

Caverhill, W.C.F., *Caverhill's Toronto City Directory for 1859-60* (Toronto: Lovell and Gibson, 1859), 282.

Chadwick, Edward Marion, "Jarvis" in *Ontarian Families* (Toronto: Rolph, Smith and Company, 1894), 127-128.

Chance, Burton, "Sir William Lawrence in relation to Medical Education with Special Reference to Ophthalmology in the Early Part of the Nineteenth Century," *Annals of Medical History*, 8 (1926), 270-279.

Charlton, M., "William Rawlins Beaumont, F.R.C.S. (Eng.) (1803-1875)," *Annals of Medical History*, 3 (1921), 284-6.

Cherrier, Kirwin and McGown's Toronto Directory for 1873 (Toronto: Cherrier, Kirwin and McGown, 1873), 34.

Chisholm, Hugh, ed., "Sewing Machines," *The Encyclopaedia Britannica, A Dictionary of Arts, Sciences, Literature and General Information* (Cambridge: University Press, 1911), 24, 744-745.

Churchill, Fleetwood, *On the Diseases of Women* (Dublin: Fannin and Co. 41, Grafton Street, 1864), 18-19.

City of York Assessment Rolls, St. George's Ward, 1844, p. 15 (#285), in City of Toronto Archives, New City Hall, Nathan Phillips Square, Toronto, Ontario, Canada.

City of York Assessment Rolls, St. George's Ward, 1845, p. 16 (#289), in City of Toronto Archives, New City Hall, Nathan Phillips Square, Toronto, Ontario.

City of York Assessment Rolls, St. George's Ward, 1846, in City of Toronto Archives, New City Hall, Nathan Phillips Square, Toronto, Ontario.

City of York Assessment Rolls, St. Patrick's Ward, 1843, p. 6 (#121), City of

Toronto Archives, New City Hall, Nathan Phillips Square, Toronto, Ontario.

Clarke, Charles K., *A History of the Toronto General Hospital* (Toronto: William Briggs, 1913),

Clarke, Edwin, "Hall, Marshall," in *D.S.B.*, 6 (1972), 58-61.

Clements, Paul, *Marc Isambard Brunel* (Harlow: Longmans, 1970).

Cook, Ramsay, Saywell, John, and Ricker, John, *Canada: A Modern Study* (Toronto: Clark, Irwin and Company, 1963).

Cooper, Bransby Blake, *The Life of Sir Astley Cooper, Bart., Interspersed with sketches from his note books of distinguished contemporary characters* (London: J.W. Parker, 1843).

Cooper, Grace Rogers, "The Invention of the Sewing Machine," *Smithsonian Institution United States National Museum, Bulletin* 254(1968).

Cornelius, Medvei Victor, and Thornton, John L., Eds., *The Royal Hospital of St. Bartholomew* (London: St. Bartholomew's Hospital Medical College, 1974).

Cosbie, W.G., *The Toronto General Hospital, 1819-1965* (Toronto: Macmillan of Canada, 1975).

Cushing, Harvey, *The Life of Sir William Osler* (1849-1919), 1-2 (New York: Oxford University Press, 1925; reprinted 1940, 1 volume).

Daumas, Maurice, *A History of Technology and Invention: Progress Through the Ages*, 3 (New York: Crown Publishers, 1979), 162-163.

Dolman, Claude E., "Bovell, James," in La Terreur, Marc, ed., Dictionary of Canadian Biography [hereafter *D.C.B.*] (Toronto: University of Toronto Press 1972), 10, 83-83.

Dunlop, William, *Tiger Dunlop's Upper Canada* (Toronto: McClelland and Stewart, 1967).

Dyster, Barrie, "Gwynne, William," *D.C.B.*, 10(1972), 325-6.

Farnie, D.A., "The Textile Industry: Woven Fabrics," in Singer, Charles, Holmyard, E.J., Hall, A. Rupert, and Williams, Trevor, ed., *A History of Technology* (Oxford: Clarendon Press, 1958), 5, 569-574.

Final report of the Commissioners of Inquiry into the Affairs of King's College University, and Upper Canada College (Quebec: Rollo Campbell, 1852).

Franklin, Kenneth J., ed. and trans., William Harvey: *The Circulation of the Blood and Other Writings* (London: Everyman's Library, 1963).

Fulton, John F., "William Osler as a Medical Historian," *University of Manitoba Medical Journal*, (Feb., 1949), 20.

Fulton, John F., and Rosen, George, *The Reception of William Beaumont's Discovery in Europe* (New York: Schuman's, 1942).

Godfrey, Charles M., "King's College: Upper Canada's First Medical School," *Ontario Medical Review*, 34(1967), 19-22.

Godfrey, Charles M., *Cholera in Upper Canada, 1832-1860* (Toronto: Seccombe House, 1968).

Godfrey, Charles, *Medicine for Ontario: a History* (Belleville: Mika Publishing Company, 1979).

H.J. Milburn and Company, *General Prices Current of Surgical Instruments and Appliances* (Detroit, Michigan: H.J. Milburn and Company, circa 1893), 52-53. In Museum of the History of Medicine, Toronto Academy of Medicine.

Hall, Charlotte, *Memoirs of Marshall Hall, M.D., F.R.S.* (London: R. Bentley, 1861).

Hambrecht, F. Terry, "The History of George Tiemann & Co., 1826-1986," *Medical Collectors Association Newsletter*, #8 (December, 1986).

Harris, Charles, "William Thomas Aikins," *Canadian Journal of Surgery*, 5(1962), 131-137.

Harvey, Alexander, "The Sewing Machine abolishes a fundamental class distinction," in Baker, Ray Stannard et al., *Modern Inventions and Discoveries* (New York: J.A. Hill and Company, 1904), 288-294.

Hirsch, August, ed., "Beaumont, William Rawlins," *Biographisches Lexikon der Hervorragenden Artze aller Zeiten und Völker* (Berlin: Urban & Schwarzenberg, 1929), 1, 404.

Hodder, Edward, "Cases of Ovariotomy," *Canada Lancet*, 4, #10 (June, 1872), 446-455.

Hodgins, J. George, ed., *Documentary History of Education in Upper Canada*, 1-10, (Toronto: Warwick Brothers and Rutter-L.K. Cameron, 1897-1903.

Howell, Thomas, "A Case of Abscess in the Groin, attended with Symptoms of Hernia, from which two Lumbrici Teretes and afterwards Faecal Matter were discharged, and the patient recovered, by Thos. Howell, Esq. of Risborough," *London Medical Gazette*, 36(1845), 35.

Hunter, Robert, "A Newly Licensed Practitioner," *Toronto Globe*, 4, #90, whole number 248 (Saturday, November 13, 1847), p. 2-3.

Hutchinson's Toronto Directory, 1862-63 (Toronto: Lovell and Gibson, 1862), 74.

Irwin, William Henry, *Robertson and Cook's Toronto City Directory for 1871-72* (Toronto: Robertson and Cook, 1871), 32.

Irwin, William Henry, *Toronto City Directory, May 1873 to May 1874* (Toronto: Hunter, Rose and Co., 1873), 28.

Jack, Donald, *Rogues, Rebels and Geniuses* (Toronto: Doubleday Canada, 1981).

Keane, David R., "Aikins, William Thomas," in Marsh, James H., ed., *The Canadian Encyclopedia,* (1988), 1, 41.

Kelly's Post Office London Business Directory, 188th Edition (East Grinstead, West Sussex: Kelly's Directories, 1987), 1, 185.

Keys, Thomas Edward, *The History of Surgical Anaesthesia* (New York: Dover Publications, 1963).

Klinck, Carl F., *William "Tiger" Dunlop: "Blackwoodian Backwoodsman"* (Toronto: The Ryerson Press, 1958).

Lacaine, A.V., and Laurent, H.C., "Amussat (Jean Zuléma)," in *Biographies et Nécrologies des hommes marquants du XIX siècle,* 1-7(Paris: 1844-1866).

Lawrence, William, *An Introduction to Comparative Anatomy and Physiology: being the Two Introductory Lectures Delivered at the Royal College of Surgeons on the 21st and 25th of March, 1816* (London: 1816).

Lawrence, William, *Lectures on the Physiology, Zoology, and the Natural History of Man, Delivered at the Royal College of Surgeons* (London: 1819; reprinted London: James Smith, 1823).

LeFanu, William, "Mayo, Herbert," in *D.S.B.,* 10(1974), 241-242.

Lewis, Francis, *The Toronto Directory and Street Guide for 1843-44* (Toronto: H. & W. Boswell, 1843), 21, 81.

Lewton, Frederick A., "The Servant in the House: A Brief History of the Sewing Machine" *Annual Report of the Smithsonian Institution* (1929), (publication 3034), 559-583.

Lilley, S., *Men, Machines and History* (New York: International Publishers, 1966).

Lizars, John Lizars, "Excision of Nearly One Half of Inferior Maxilla," *Canada Lancet,* 5, #2 (Oct., 1872), 57-60.

Macara, John, *Letters on King's College by the Rev. John McCaul* (Toronto: Examiner Office, 1848).

Macara, John, *The Origin, History and Management of the University of King's College, Toronto* (Toronto: George Brown, 1844), 66-67.

Macilwain, George, *Memoirs of John Abernethy: with a view of his lectures, writings and character* (London: Hatchel, 1856).

Mayo, Herbert, *Anatomical and Physiological Commentaries*, Part 1 (London: Thomas and George Underwood,1822); Part 2 (London: Thomas and George Underwood, 1823).

McEvoy, Henry, C.E. *Anderson and Co. Toronto City Directory for 1868-69* (Toronto: C.E. Anderson, 1868), 165, 190, 373.

McKinney, H. Lewis, "Lawrence, William," in *D.S.B.*, 8(1973), 96-98.

McNaught, Kenneth, *The Pelican History of Canada* (Markham, Ontario: Penguin Books Canada, 1976), 129, 148-149.

McNeil, Chester, *A History of the Sewing Machine* (Chicago: Union Special Sewing Machine Company, 1903).

Medical Faculty, *Church University* (Toronto: A.F. Plees, 1851), 6-7.

Medvei, Victor Cornelius, and Thornton, John L., eds., *The Royal Hospital of St. Bartholomew* (London: W.S. Cowell, 1974).

Melville, Henry, *The Rise and Progress of Trinity College, Toronto* (Toronto: Henry Rowsell, 1852), 168-169.

Middleton, Jesse Edgar, *"Institutions of Higher Learning," in The Municipality of Toronto: A History* (Toronto: Dominion Publishing Company, 1923), 2, 571-588.

Minutes of Meetings of Corporation Minute Book, 7 July 1868-22 April 1887 (Medical School of Trinity College), 32-33 (Wednesday, March 8, 1871); in *Corporation Minute Book 986-001/013*, Trinity College Archives, Trinity College, University of Toronto, Toronto, Ontario, Canada.

Mitchell and Co.'s *General Directory for the City of Toronto, and Gazeteer of the Counties of York and Peel for 1866* (Toronto: Mitchell and Co., 1866), 185.

Mitchell's Toronto Directory for 1864-5 (Toronto: W.C. Chewett, 1864), 83.

Morton, W.L., *The Kingdom of Canada: A General History from Earliest Times* (Toronto: McClelland and Stewart, 1980), 322-323.

Müller, Johannes, and Schwan, Theodore, "Versuche über die künstliche

Mitchell's Toronto Directory for 1864-5 (Toronto: W.C. Chewett, 1864), 83.

Morton, W.L., *The Kingdom of Canada: A General History from Earliest Times* (Toronto: McClelland and Stewart, 1980), 322-323.

Müller, Johannes, and Schwan, Theodore, "Versuche über die künstliche Verdauung des geronnenen Eiweisses," *Archiv für Anatomie und Physiologie*, (1836), 66-89.

Mumford, Lewis, *Technics and Civilization* (New York: Harcourt, Brace and World, 1934; reprinted 1963), 92-93.

Myer, Jesse S., *The Life and Letters of Dr. William Beaumont Including Hitherto Unpublished Data Concerning the Case of Alexis St. Martin* (St. Louis: C.V. Mosby, 1912; reprinted 1939).

Ontario Genealogical Society, Toronto Branch, *Cathedral Church of St. James (Anglican) Marriages, 1800-1908*, p. 381 (fiche #4), record #4386, in St. James Anglican Cathedral Church Archives, 131 Adelaide Street East, Toronto, Ontario.

Ontario Genealogical Society, Toronto Branch, *Register of Baptisms, 1807-1908: St. James Cathedral, Toronto*; Register 3, p. 198 (fiche #8), record #3-2227, in St. James Anglican Cathedral Archives, 131 Adelaide Street East, Toronto, Ontario.

Ontario Genealogical Society, Toronto Branch, *St. James Cathedral, Toronto — Index of Baptisms — 1807 to 1908*; Register 3, p. 17, (fiche #6), St. James Anglican Cathedral archives, 131 Adelaide Street East, Toronto, Ontario.

Ontario Genealogical Society, Toronto Branch, *St. James Cathedral, Toronto — Index of Baptisms — 1807 to 1908*; Register 4, p. 102, record #1142, in St. James' Anglican Cathedral Archives, 131 Adelaide Street East, Toronto, Ontario.

Osler, William, *Aequanimitas: With other Addresses to Medical Students, Nurses and Practitioners of Medicine* (London: H.K. Lewis, 1904), 175-176, 369.

Paget, James, *St. Bartholomew's Hospital and School Fifty Years Ago* (London: Medical Magazine Association, 1905), 29.

Paget, Sir James, "William Rawlins Beaumont," *Proceedings of the Royal Medical and Chirurgical Society*, 8 (1875-80), 72.

Paget, Stephen, *Memoirs and Letters of Sir James Paget* (London: Longman, Green and Company, 1903), 45-46.

Patten, James, "Sewing Machines," *The Encyclopedia Britannica*, (Chicago: R.S. Peale Company, 1892), 21, 718-720.

Pilon, Henri, "Hodder, Edward Mulberry," *D.C.B.*, 10 (1972), 350-351.

Power, D'Arcy, ed., *Plarr's Lives of the Fellows of the Royal College of Surgeons of England*, 1- 2 (London: Simpkin Marshall, 1930).

Pursell, Carroll W., "Machines and Machine Tools," in Kranzberg, Melvin and Pursell, Carroll W., ed., *Technology in Western Civilization*, 1 (New York: Oxford University Press, 1967), 403-404.

Pursell, Carroll, "Technology in America: An Introduction," in Pursell, Carroll, ed., *Technology in America: A History of Individuals and Ideas* (Cambridge, Mass: MIT Press, 1982).

Reed, T.A., ed., *A History of the University of Trinity College* (Toronto: University of Toronto Press, 1952), 76.

Reeve, Richard A., "A Case of Foreign Body in the Orbit, with Remarks," *Canada Lancet*, 4, #1 (September, 1871), 15-19.

Report of an Investigation by the Trustees of the Toronto General Hospital into Certain Charges Against the Management of that Institution (Toronto: Globe Book and Job Office, 22 King Street West, 1855).

Richardson, James, "Reminisces of Dr. James H. Richardson," (April, 1905), unpublished typescript, "Baldwin Room," Metro Toronto Reference Library, Toronto, Ontario, p. 7.

Richardson, James, letter to Loudon, James, June 27, 1899, in James Loudon Papers, R23, B72- 0031/008, Q-Sou, University of Toronto Archives, Toronto, Ontario.

Roberts, Shirley, *Sir James Paget: The Rise of Clinical Surgery* (London: Royal Society of Medicine Services Limited, 1989).

Robertson, J. Ross, *Landmarks of Toronto, A Collection of Historical Sketches of the Old Town of York* (Toronto: J. Ross Robertson, 1898; reprinted Belleville, Ontario: Mika Publishing, 1974).

Roland, Charles, "Medicine, History of," in Marsh, James H., ed., *The Canadian Encyclopedia*, 2 (Edmonton: Hurtig Publishers, 1988), 1329.

Rolph, John, *Address of the Honourable Dr. Rolph delivered before the Faculty and Students of Medicine of the University of Victoria College, Toronto, 1854-5* (Toronto: T. H. Bentley, 1855).

Rolph, John, "Introductory Lecture of the Hon. John Rolph delivered before the Faculty and Students of Medicine of the University of Victoria College, Toronto, Session 1860-61" (Toronto: The Guardian, 1861).

Romney, Paul, "Widmer, Christopher," in *D.C.B.*, 8, (1985), 931-936.

Rosen, George, "Beaumont, William [1785-1853]," D.S.B., 1, (1970), 542-545.

Schwann, Theodore, "Ueber das Wesen der Verdauungsprocesses" *Archiv für Anatomie und Physiologie*, (1836), 90-138.

Sieveking, Paul, ed., *British Biographical Archive* (London: K.G. Saur, 1984).

Spear, Robert, *An Essay on Madness; Containing the Outlines of a New Theory* (Toronto: H. and W. Rowsell, 1844).

Spear, Robert, *Introduction to an Essay on Science* (Toronto: H. and W. Rowsell, 1844).

St. James (Anglican) Cathedral Cemetery, Register of Burials, Reel 1, (June 1844-June 1879), p. 162; in St. James Cathedral Church Archives, 131 Adelaide Street East, Toronto, Ontario.

St. James' Cemetery, Toronto: Register of Internments: (May, 1931), "Charlotte Jarvis," Interment Number 47443, (Reel #1: January 1930-May, 1957), in St. James' Anglican Cathedral Archives, 131 Adelaide Street East, Toronto, Ontario.

Starr, F.N.G., "President's Address — 'The Passing of the Surgeon' in Toronto," President's address at the opening meeting (October 3, 1901) of the Toronto Medical Society; reprinted in the *Canadian Practitioner and Review*, 26, #12 (December, 1901), 666.

Strachan, John, letter to Beaumont, William, January 18, 1848; in *Letter Book 6*, p. 272, in Strachan Papers, MS 35, v. 12, 7-430, Ontario Government Archives, 77 Grenville Street, Toronto, Ontario.

Stratford, Samuel, "Rough notes of a clinical lecture, delivered by Dr. Beaumont, F.R.C.S. London, and one of the surgeons to the Toronto General Hospital, on a case of false aneurysm. Reported from memory," *Upper Canada Journal of Medical, Surgical, and Physical Science*, 3 (1853-54), 251-8.

Sutherland, James, *City of Toronto Directory for 1867-8* (Toronto: W.C. Chewett, 1867), 147.

The British Library General Catalogue of Printed Books to 1975, 22 (London: Clive Bingley, 1979), 302.

Thompson, C.J.S., *Guide to the Surgical Instruments and Objects in the Historical Series with their History and Development*. (London: Royal College of Surgeons of England Museum, 1929).

Thompson, C.J.S., *Lord Lister, the Discoverer of Antiseptic Surgery* (London: Bale, Sons and Danielsson, 1934);

Thompson, C.J.S., *The History and Evolution of Surgical Instruments* (New York: Schuman's, 1942).

Toronto Directory for 1877 (Toronto: Might and Taylor, 1877), 454-5, 493, 513.

Toronto Directory for 1878 (Toronto: Might and Taylor, 1878), 229.

Toronto Directory for 1880 (Toronto: Might and Taylor, 1880), 49 209.

Toronto Globe, 23, #213 (September 5, 1866), whole number 5129, p. 2.

Townsend, P.S., editor and translator, *Alfred A. L. M. Velpeau's New Elements of Operative Surgery* (New York: Samuel S. and William Wood, 1847), 1, 724.

University of Trinity College Toronto School of Medicine Annual Announcement (T 2.2), Box P 78-0069 to -0070 [P78-0070(.03)], University of Toronto Archives, Toronto, Ontario, Canada.

University of Trinity College Toronto School of Medicine Annual Announcement (T 2.2), Box P 78-0069 to -0070 [P78-0070(.04)], University of Toronto Archives, Toronto, Ontario, Canada.

Vaperau, L.G., "Amussat (Jean Zuléma)," *Dictionnaire universel des Contemporains* (Paris: Hachette & cie, 1893).

Walker, Kenneth, *Joseph Lister* (London: Hutchinson, 1956).

Wallace, William Stewart, *A History of the University of Toronto, 1827-1927* (Toronto: University of Toronto Press, 1927).

Wallace, William Stewart, "Sullivan, Robert Baldwin," in *The Encyclopedia of Canada* (Toronto: University Associates, 1948), 6, 81.

Wallace, William Stewart, "Fenian Raids," (1948), 2, 328-329.

Wallace, William Stewart, "O'Brien, Lucius James" (1948), 5, 37.

Wallace, William Stewart, "Workman, Joseph," (1948), 6, 322.

Wallace, William Stewart, "Hincks, Sir Francis," (1948), 3, 142.

Wallace, William Stewart, "Workman, Joseph," *The Macmillan Dictionary of Canadian Biography* (Toronto: Macmillan, 1978), 906.

Wangensteen, Owen H., and Wangensteen, Sarah D., *The Rise of Surgery: from Empiric Craft to Scientific Discipline* (Minneapolis: University of Minnesota Press, 1987) 537-538.

Weinreb, Ben, and Hibbert, Christopher, eds., *The London Encyclopedia* (London: Macmillan, 1983).

Welton, Thurston Scott, "Biographical Brevities: William Rawlins Beaumont," *The American Journal of Surgery*, New Series, 28, #1 (April, 1935), 182.

West, Bruce, *Toronto* (Toronto: Doubleday, 1967).

Whitney, William, ed., "Sewing Machine," *The Century Dictionary*, (New York: The Century Company, 1906).

Wilbur, C. Keith, *Antique Medical Instruments* (West Chester, Pennsylvania: Schiffer Publishing Ltd., 1987).

York County Toronto Surrogate Court Records: Wills. #2090 in roll 1984-2099 (covering period 1873-1876), (G.S. Ont. 1-975) 2-438 at the Ontario Government Archives, 77 Grenville Street, Toronto, Ontario.

Publications by Doctor William Beaumont

Beaumont, William, "A Description of a new Instrument for Closing Vesico-Vaginal and Recto-Vaginal Fistulae, and Fissures of the Soft Palate," *Medico-Chirurgical Transactions*, 21(Second Series, 3), (1838), 29-32, plus figure 1.

Beaumont, William, "Apparatus for making Extension in Fractures of the Lower Extremity of the Radius," Upper Canada Journal of Medical, Surgical and Physical Sciences, 2 (1852-1853), 126- 127; 157-158.

Beaumont, William, "Case of Disarticulation of the Left Condyle of the Lower Jaw" *Medico-Chirurgical Transactions*, 33 (Second Series, 15), 1850, 243-248.

Beaumont, William, "Case of Lithotomy," *Braithwaite's Retrospect of Practical Medicine and Surgery*, 34 (January, 1857), 115-116.

Beaumont, William, "Case of Strangulated Hernia, Insidiously Fatal," *London Medical Gazette*, 14 (Saturday, July 12, 1834), 525-526.

Beaumont, William, "Case of Traumatic Carotid Aneurism," *Braithwaite's Retrospect of Practical Medicine and Surgery*, 30 (January, 1855), 130.

Beaumont, William, "Cases of Operation for Cataract," *Upper Canada*

Journal of Medical, Surgical and Physical Science, 2 (1852-1853), 177-179.

Beaumont, William, "Cases of Operations for Cataract, Chiefly at the Toronto General Hospital," *Upper Canada Journal of Medical, Surgical and Physical Science,* 1 (1851-1852), 329-332, 361-365, 407-411, 510-515.

Beaumont, William, "Cases of Stone in the Bladder — Lithotrity," *Canada Lancet,* 3, #1 (September, 1870), 35-37.

Beaumont, William, "Cheiloplasty, and Operation for Atresia Oris," *Upper Canada Journal of Medical, Surgical and Physical Science,* 1 (1851-1852), 54-59.

Beaumont, William, "Clinical Lecture on a Case of Traumatic Carotid Aneurism," *Lancet,* (July 29, 1854), 75-78.

Beaumont, William, "Clinical Lecture on a Deeply Penetrating Wound of the Head, by a Rocket- Shaft Passing through the Left Orbit," *Lancet,* (June 14, 1862), 626-627.

Beaumont, William, "Clinical Lecture on the Several Forms of Lithotomy," *Lancet* (January 24, 1857), 81-2.

Beaumont, William, "Description of a New Iris Forceps," *Medico-Chirurgical Transactions,* 46 (Second Series, 28), (1863), 175-180.

Beaumont, William, "Description of a New Iris Forceps," *Lancet,* (June 27, 1863), 718.

Beaumont, William, "Dr. Beaumont's Case of Aneurism," *Upper Canada Journal of Medical, Surgical and Physical Science,* 3 (1853-1854), 325-327.

Beaumont, William, "Exostosis of Scapula," *London Medical Gazette,* 23 (Saturday, October 27, 1838), 162-163.

Beaumont, William, "Instrument for Closing Recto-Vaginal or Vesico-Vaginal Fistulae," *London Medical Gazette,* 19 (Saturday, December 3, 1836), 335.

Beaumont, William, "Laceration of Internal Parts, without Internal Lesion," *London Medical Gazette,* 15 (Saturday, February 21, 1835), 727-728.

Beaumont, William, "Last Will and Testament," *York County, Toronto Surrogate Court: Wills.* Number 2090 in roll for 1984-2099, covering years 1873-1876 (G.S. Ont. 1-975); microfilm 2- 438 at Ontario Government Archives, 77 Grenville Street, Toronto, Ontario, Canada.

Beaumont, William, "New Speculum Vaginae," *London Medical Gazette,* 20 (Saturday, April 27, 1837), 122-123.

Beaumont, William, "Treatment of Fractures by Means of Plaster of Paris," *London Medical Gazette*, 21 (Saturday, January 6, 1838), 589-90.

Beaumont, William, "Two Cases of Formation of Artificial Pupil, with the description of a new Instrument for seizing and detaching the Iris, by W. R. Beaumont," *London Medical Gazette*, 36 (1845), 33-34.

Beaumont, William, *An Account of Some New Instruments for tying Polypi of the Uterus, Nose and Ear, and Enlarged Tonsils, with Cases* (London: J. Churchill, 1838).

Beaumont, William, letter to Baldwin, Robert, April 26, 1849, A33-#81, *Robert Baldwin Papers*, "Baldwin Room," Metro Toronto Research Library, Toronto, Ontario.

Beaumont, William, *Observations and Experiments on a New Mode of Treating Fractures of the Leg and Fore-Arm; Especially Compound Fractures* (London: Longmans, 1831).

NOTES AND REFERENCES

1. "Mr. William Smith O'Brien in Toronto," *The Daily Globe*, 16, #107 (whole number 2,832), (Thursday, May 5, 1859), 3; "The Rocket Accident on Wednesday Evening," *The Daily Globe*, 16, #108 (whole number 2,833), (Friday, May 6, 1859), 3.
2. Osler, William, *Aequanimitas: With other Addresses to Medical Students, Nurses and Practitioners of Medicine* (London: H.K. Lewis, 1904), 175–176, 369.
3. Thompson, C.J.S., *The History and Evolution of Surgical Instruments* (New York: Schuman's, 1942).
4. Keys, Thomas Edward, *The History of Surgical Anaesthesia* (New York: Dover Publications, 1963).
5. Thompson, C.J.S., *Lord Lister, the Discoverer of Antiseptic Surgery* (London: Bale, Sons and Danielsson, 1934); Walker, Kenneth, *Joseph Lister* (London: Hutchinson, 1956).
6. Roland, Charles, "Medicine, History of", in Marsh, James H., ed., *The Canadian Encyclopedia*, 2 (Edmonton: Hurtig Publishers, 1988), 1329.
7. Boase, F., ed., "Beaumont, William Rawlins", in *Modern English Biography*, 1–6 (Truro: For the Author, 1892–1921; reprinted London: F. Cass, 1965); also reprinted in Sieveking, Paul, ed., *British Biographical Archive* (London: K.G. Saur, 1984). See also "The Late Dr. Beaumont", *Canada Lancet*, 8, #3 (November 1, 1875), 92–93; and "Obituary: William Rawlins Beaumont, M.D., F.R.C.S. Eng.", *British Medical Journal*, 2 (December 11, 1875), 749–750.
8. Jack, Donald, *Rogues, Rebels and Geniuses* (Toronto: Doubleday Canada, 1981), 72.
9. Jack mentions some of these instruments, but emphasizes the deep-suturing tool and, like many other historians, says it was the inspiration for the sewing machine. If this is true, it is of enormous importance to the history of technology, for the critical role of the sewing machine in revolutionizing industry and bringing the "American system of mass manufacturing" into the home has long been realized. See Pursell, Carroll, "Technology in America: An Introduction", in Pursell, Carroll, ed., *Technology in America: A History of Individuals and Ideas* (Cambridge, Mass.: The MIT Press, 1982), 3.

10. Charlton, M., "William Rawlins Beaumont, F.R.C.S. (Eng.) (1803–1875)," *Annals of Medical History*, 3 (1921), 284–6.
11. Most sources say simply that he received a "liberal education" or a "sound preliminary education." See, for example, "Obituary – William R. Beaumont, F.R.C.S., Eng.," *Canada Medical and Surgical Journal*, 4 (1876), 238–240, p. 239; "Obituary, William Rawlins Beaumont, M.D., F.R.C.S. Eng.," *British Medical Journal*, 2 (1875), 749–750, p. 749.
12. For more on Harvey, see Bylebyl, Jerome J., "Harvey, William," in Gillespie, Charles Coulston, ed., *Dictionary of Scientific Biography* (New York: Charles Scribner's Sons, 1972) [hereafter D.S.B.], 6, 150–162; and Franklin, Kenneth J., ed. and trans., *William Harvey: The Circulation of the Blood and Other Writings* (London: Everyman's Library, 1963).
13. For more on Abernethy, see Macilwain, George, *Memoirs of John Abernethy: with a view of his lectures, writings and character* (London: Hatchel, 1856).
14. Charlton, M., 284
15. "Obituary – William R. Beaumont, F.R.C.S., Eng.", *Canada Medical and Surgical Journal*, 4 (1876), 239. See also "The Late Dr. Beaumont", *Canada Lancet*, 8, #3 (November 1, 1875), 92–3, and Charlton, 284.
16. Beaumont, William, "Clinical Lecture on a Deeply Penetrating Wound of the Head, by a Rocket–Shaft Passing through the Left Orbit," *Lancet*, (June 14, 1862), 626–627. There is no obstruction to the passage of a thin stick or projectile into the brain through the eye socket. Sometimes the object can tear the intracranial carotid artery on the way, with fatal results.
17. Paget, James, *St. Bartholomew's Hospital and School Fifty Years Ago* (London: The Medical Magazine Association, 1905), 29.
18. Paget, James, (1905), 29. Charles Simeon (1759–1836) was educated at Eton and King's College, Cambridge, and in 1783 became the perpetual curate at Cambridge's Holy Trinity Church.
19. Beaumont, William, "Laceration of Internal Parts, without Internal Lesion", *London Medical Gazette*, 15 (Saturday, February 21, 1835), 727–728.
20. Beaumont, William, "Laceration of Internal Parts", 728. Beaumont's description of "a sound as of air rushing through the wound" is consistent with what is today referred to as "tension pneumothorax."

Following the puncture of the pleural membrane and the underlying lung by a broken rib, air passes from the lung to the pleural cavity where, unable to escape, it builds up. The lung is collapsed by the accumulated air in the pleural cavity and, if not released, is often fatal. It is not clear why the patient in this case died as soon as the trapped air was released.

21. For more on Cooper, see Cooper, Bransby Blake, *The Life of Sir Astley Cooper, Bart., Interspersed with sketches from his note-books of distinguished contemporary characters* (London: J.W. Parker, 1843).
22. Mayo, Herbert, *Anatomical and Physiological Commentaries*, (London: Thomas and George Underwood. Part 1 1822; Part 2, 1823).
23. For more on Mayo, see LeFanu, William, "Mayo, Herbert," in D.S.B., 10 (1974), 241–242, and Power, D'Arcy, ed., Parr's *Lives of the Fellows of the Royal College of Surgeons of England* (London: Simpkin Marshall, 1930).
24. Lawrence, William, *An Introduction to Comparative Anatomy and Physiology: being the Two Introductory Lectures Delivered at the Royal College of Surgeons on the 21st and 25th of March, 1816* (London: 1816); *Lectures on the Physiology, Zoology, and the Natural History of Man, Delivered at the Royal College of Surgeons*(London: 1819; reprinted London: James Smith, 1823).
25. For more on Lawrence, see McKinney, H. Lewis, "Lawrence, William," in D.S.B., 8(1973), 96–98, and Chance, Burton, "Sir William Lawrence in relation to Medical Education with Special Reference to Ophthalmology in the Early Part of the Nineteenth Century," *Annals of Medical History*, 8 (1926), 270–279.
26. Paget, Stephen, *Memoirs and Letters of Sir James Paget*(London: Longman, Green and Company, 1903), 45–46.
27. Bell, Gary, "William Rawlins Beaumont 1803–1875: An Inventor Surgeon," *Bulletin of the Academy of Medicine, Toronto*, 50, #3 (March, 1977), 49–51, names this figure as Jean–Andre Amussat. They are the same. Lacaine, A.V., and Laurent, H.C., "Amussat (Jean Zuléma)," in *Biographies et Nécrologies des hommes marquants du XIX siècle*, 1–7(Paris: 1844–1866); Vaperau, L.G., "Amussat (Jean Zuléma)," *Dictionnaire universel des Contemporains*(Paris: Hachette & cie., 1893).
28. "Obituary, William Rawlins Beaumont, M.D., F.R.C.S. Eng.," *British Medical Journal*, 2 (1875), 749–750. Charlton, Ibid., 285, and others say December 23, 1826, but Power, D'Arcy, (1930), 1, 73–75, confirms the December 22 date.

29. For more on Hall, see Clarke, Edwin, "Hall, Marshall," in D.S.B.,6 (1972), 58–61, and Hall, Charlotte, Memoirs of Marshall Hall, M.D., F.R.S.(London: 1861).
30. Beaumont, William, *Observations and Experiments on a New Mode of Treating Fractures of the Leg and Fore–Arm; Especially Compound Fractures*(London: Longmans, 1831). This work is summarized in Wangensteen, Owen H., and Wangensteen, Sarah D., *The Rise of Surgery: from Empiric Craft to Scientific Discipline*(Minneapolis: University of Minnesota Press, 1987) 537–538. See also Beaumont, William, "Treatment of Fractures by Means of Plaster of Paris," *London Medical Gazette*, 21(Saturday, January 6, 1838), 589–90, and "Mr. Beaumont on Fractures", *Medico–Chirurgical Review, New Series*, 16 (January 1, 1832), 247–51, p. 248. Beaumont's surmise about the healing of fractures was proved correct in World War II in the North Africa campaign. When the Eighth Army was under siege at Tobruk by Rommel, replenishment of medical supplies was cut off. A compound fracture of the leg was then treated by immobilization (in a Thomas splint) and covering with dressing and plaster of paris. The stink of putrefaction was overpowering and the abundance of maggots inside the dressing and plaster alarming. But the treatment was so beneficial that some civilian casualties were later treated the same way.
31. "Mr. Beaumont on Fractures," 247–51. The inflammatory reaction is the fundamental phenomenon of all wound healing, and the redness, swelling and pain were evidence of repair, but this was not clear in Beaumont's day.
32. Beaumont, William, "Treatment of Fractures," 589.
33. *London Medical and Surgical Journal*, October 1831; this is quoted in Beaumont, William, "Treatment of Fractures", Ibid., 589.
34. Beaumont, William, "Case of Strangulated Hernia, Insidiously Fatal", *London Medical Gazette*, 14 (Saturday, July 12, 1834), 525–526.
35. Canniff, William, *The Medical Profession in Upper Canada, 1783–1850*(Toronto: William Briggs, 1894; reprinted Toronto: Clarke, Irwin and Co., 1981), 243.
36. There appears to be some uncertainty about these instruments. Two of them, the vaginal fistula and deep-seated suturing tools, have both been variously claimed as the original inspiration for the sewing machine. These competing arguments will be examined in

more detail later. As for the instruments today, many still survive at the Museum of the Royal College of Surgeons in London, England; his suture instrument is numbered D34, the vaginal fistula instrument is labelled D19A, and a lithotomy knife from a later period is listed as G106 and 8. See Power, D'Arcy, Ibid., 73–74, and Thompson, C.J.S., *Guide to the Surgical Instruments and Objects in the Historical Series with their History and Development*. (London: Royal College of Surgeons of England Museum, 1929), 12. Until the 1930s, it was doubted if any of Beaumont's instruments survived in Canada; see Clarke, Charles K., *A History of the Toronto General Hospital*(Toronto: William Briggs, 1913), 104; Charlton, Ibid., 284; and Welton, Thurston Scott, "Biographical Brevities: William Rawlins Beaumont," *The American Journal of Surgery, New Series*, 28, #1 (April 1935), 182.

37. Thompson, C.J.S., The History and Evolution of Surgical Instruments(New York: Schuman's, 1942), 52–53; Wilbur, C. Keith, *Antique Medical Instruments*(West Chester, Pennsylvania: Schiffer Publishing Ltd., 1987), 68–69.

38. Churchill, Fleetwood, *On the Diseases of Women*(Dublin: Fannin and Co. 41, Grafton Street, 1864), 18–19.

39. "Royal Medical and Chirurgical Society, Tuesday, March 14, 1837", *London Medical Gazette*, 19 (Saturday, March 18, 1837), 938–939.

40. Beaumont, William, *An Account of Some New Instruments for tying Polypi of the Uterus, Nose and Ear, and Enlarged Tonsils, with Cases* (London: J. Churchill, 1838). This book is now very rare. The University of Toronto library had a copy in the 1850s (probably a gift from Beaumont), according to the *Alphabetical Catalogue of the Library of the University of Toronto* (Toronto: Henry Roswell, 1857), 16. But it is no longer there; it may have been lost, stolen, or destroyed by fire. Copies do survive in the British Museum Library and the Bibliothèque Nationale. See *The British Library General Catalogue of Printed Books to 1975*, 22 (London: Clive Bingley, 1979), 302, and *Catalogue Général des Livres Imprimés de la Bibliothèque Nationale: Auteurs*, 9 (Paris: Imprimerie Nationale, 1902), 513.

41. Beaumont, William, "Exostosis of Scapula," *London Medical Gazette*, 23(Saturday, October 27, 1838), 162–163.

42. For more on Widmer, see Romney, Paul, "Widmer, Christopher," in La Terreur, Marc, ed., *Dictionary of Canadian Biography* [hereafter

D.C.B.] (Toronto: University of Toronto Press, 1985), 8, 931–936; see also Canniff, William, (1894), 656–663. For Widmer's loyalty to Beaumont, see Romney, Paul, (1985), 8, 933– 934.

43. Dyster, Barrie, "Gwynne, William," D.C.B., 10(1972), 325–326.
44. Canniff, William, (1894), 668–672; Wallace, William Stewart, "Workman, Joseph," *The Macmillan Dictionary of Canadian Biography* (Toronto: Macmillan, 1978), 906.
45. "Licentiates of the Medical Board of Upper Canada," *The British American Journal of Medical and Physical Science*, 3(1847–1848), 250.
46. Ontario Genealogical Society, Toronto Branch, *St. James Cathedral, Toronto — Index of Baptisms* — 1807 to 1908; Register 3, p. 17 (fiche #6), in St. James Anglican Cathedral Archives, 131 Adelaide Street East, Toronto, Ontario.
47. Godfrey, Charles M., "King's College: Upper Canada's First Medical School," *Ontario Medical Review*, 34(1967), 19–22; Canniff, William, (1894), 183–186; Hodgins, J. George, ed., *Documentary History of Education in Upper Canada*, 4 (1841–1843), (Toronto: Warwick Brothers and Rutter, 1897), 293–299; "Minutes of the Proceedings of the Council of King's College at a meeting held on the 25th day of September, 1843," *King's College Council Minute Book*, III(Nov. 1842–Dec. 1848), 19–20, in Board of Governors, A70–0024, in University of Toronto Archives, Toronto, Ontario. By 1845 Beaumont was receiving £222.4s.5d.a year from King's College for his two-term course in surgery. See the *Final Report of the Commissioners of Inquiry into the Affairs of King's College University and Upper Canada College*(Quebec: Rollo Campbell, 1852), 109.
48. Godfrey, Charles, *Medicine for Ontario*(Belleville, Ontario: Mika, 1979), 50; Boys, Henry, "University of King's College, Toronto: Hilary Term, 1844," *British Colonist*, 8, #2, (whole number 333), (Tuesday, January 9, 1844), page 3.
49. Richardson, James, "Reminiscences of Dr. James H. Richardson," (April, 1905), unpublished typescript, "Baldwin Room," Metro Toronto Reference Library, Toronto, Ontario, p. 7.

Richardson's version of this story is almost identical to his account on page 3 of a June 27, 1899, letter to University of Toronto President James Loudon: "During the session of 1843–44, I was the sole regular attendant on Prof. Beaumont's lectures, delivered in the old Parliament buildings, and at his kind suggestion I would draw up my chair beside his, in front of the fireplace, while he read his carefully prepared lecture." For this letter, see James Loudon papers, R23, B72-0031/008, Q-Sou, University of Toronto Archives, Toronto, Ontario.

See also Richardson, James, (1905), 5–6; Richardson, letter to Loudon, (June 27, 1899), pages 2–3: "Beaumont, Professor of Surgery, Fellow of the Royal College of Surgeons, London, was pre-eminently distinguished for his professional attainments. During over 50 years of professional life I have had abundant opportunity of forming a judgment as to the skill of surgeons, not only here but during my studies for three years at London and Paris, and I unhesitatingly state that, in my opinion, Prof. Beaumont would favourably compare with the most eminent of them, in his knowledge of the principles of surgery, and as an operator."

50. Jack, Donald, *Rogues, Rebels and Geniuses*(Toronto: Doubleday Canada, 1981), 69–72; Canniff, William, (1894), 590–603; Godfrey, Charles, (1979), 73–82; Rolph, John, *Address of the Honourable Dr. Rolph delivered before the Faculty and Students of Medicine of the University of Victoria College, Toronto, 1854–5*(Toronto: T. H. Bentley, 1855); Rolph, John, *Introductory Lecture of the Hon. John Rolph delivered before the Faculty and Students of Medicine of the University of Victoria College, Toronto, Session 1860–61*(Toronto: The Guardian, 1861).
51. Canniff, William, (1894), 432–434; Pilon, Henri, "Hodder, Edward Mulberry," D.C.B., 10(1972), 350–351.
52. Godfrey, Charles, (1979), 51–52.
53. Aikins, William Thomas, loose leaf scrap book on medical education in Upper Canada at the Academy of Medicine, Toronto, Ontario, Canada. Quoted by Spragge, George W., "The Trinity Medical College", *Ontario History*, 58, #2 (June, 1966), 72.
54. Canniff, William, (1894), 36–37.
55. Canniff, William, (1894), 192.
56. Beaumont, William, "Cases of Operations for Cataract, Chiefly at the Toronto General Hospital," *Upper Canada Journal of Medical, Surgical and Physical Science*, 1(1851–1852), 329–332, 361–365, 407–411, 510–515. See pages 329–330 for Strother's case.
57. Beaumont, William, "Cataract," 331–332. Jean Pierre Maunoir (1768–1861) was a Swiss surgeon and ophthalmologist whose instruments Beaumont admired greatly. He used them a great deal.

Jacques Daviel (1696–1762) was a French ophthalmologist, who had first developed the method of treating cataracts by removing the lens.

58. Beaumont, William, "Cataract," 332. Antonio Scarpa (1747–1832) was an Italian surgeon who was celebrated for both his instruments and his work on the anatomy of the ear, nerve ganglia and bones.
59. Beaumont, William, "Cataract," 332.
60. "Two Cases of Formation of Artificial Pupil, with the description of a new Instrument for seizing and detaching the Iris, by W. R. Beaumont," *London Medical Gazette*, 36 (1845), 33–34.
61. "Correspondence: The University of Toronto and the Medical Profession of Western Canada", *British American Journal of Medical and Physical Science*, 6 (1850–1851), 42–44, 140–141, 189–191, 285–286, especially p. 286. See also Canniff, William, (1894), 194–195.
62. Sewell, S.E., letter to Widmer, Christopher, May 5, 1847; reprinted in Canniff, William, (1894), 198.
63. Hunter, Robert, letter to Henwood, Edwin, November 24, 1847; quoted in Canniff, William, (1894), 201.
64. "King's College, Toronto," *The British Journal of Medical and Physical Science*, 3(1847–1848), 25.
65. Beaumont, William, "Cataract," 407.
66. Beaumont, William, "Cataract," 408.
67. Beaumont, William, "Cataract," 410.
68. John Strachan, letter to William Beaumont, January 18, 1848; in Letter Book 6, p. 272, in Strachan Papers, MS 35, v. 12, 7–430, Ontario Government Archives, 77 Grenville Street, Toronto, Ontario.
69. Canniff, William, (1894), 203.
70. Dolman, Claude E., "Bovell, James," in D.C.B., 10(1972), 83–83; Canniff, William, (1894), 257–258.
71. Keane, David R., "Aikins, William Thomas," in Marsh, James, (1988), 1, 41.
72. Beaumont, William, "Cataracts," 510.
73. Hodgins, J. George, ed., *Documentary History of Education in Upper Canada*, 7 (Toronto: L.K. Cameron, 1901), 242-5; 8, 22–23.
74. Bell, Kenneth, "Education, Secondary and University: Ryerson and Secondary Education" in Shortt, Adam and Doughty, Arthur G., eds., *Canada and its Provinces: A History of the Canadian People and their Institutions*, 18(Toronto: T. and A. Constable, 1914), 372– 373.

75. Robertson, J. Ross, *Landmarks of Toronto, A Collection of Historical Sketches of the Old Town of York* (Toronto: J. Ross Robertson, 1898; reprinted Belleville, Ontario: Mika Publishing, 1974), 3, 7.
76. *Medical Faculty, Church University* (Toronto: A.F. Plees, 1851), 6–7; Spragge, George, (1966), 66, 98.
77. Spragge, George, (1966), 75; Melville, Henry, *The Rise and Progress of Trinity College, Toronto* (Toronto: Henry Rowsell, 1852), 168–169.
78. Beaumont, William, "Case of Disarticulation," 244.
79. Stratford, Samuel, "Rough notes of a clinical lecture, delivered by Dr. Beaumont, F.R.C.S. London, and one of the surgeons to the Toronto General Hospital, on a case of false aneurysm. Reported from memory," *Upper Canada Journal of Medical, Surgical and Physical Science*, 3 (1853–1854), 251–258.
80. Beaumont, William, "Apparatus for making Extension in Fractures of the Lower Extremity of the Radius," *Upper Canada Journal of Medical, Surgical and Physical Sciences*, 2 (1852–1853), 126–127; 157–158.
81. "Meeting of Medical Practitioners", *Upper Canada Journal of Medical, Surgical and Physical Sciences*, 2 (1852–1853), 107–112; Romney, Paul, (1985), 8, 933–934.
82. "The Act of Incorporation," *Upper Canada Journal of Medical, Surgical and Physical Sciences*, 2(1852–1853), 167–174; Romney, Paul, (1985), 8, 933–934.
83. Beaumont, William, "Clinical Lecture on a Case of Traumatic Carotid Aneurism," *Lancet*, (July 29, 1854), 75–78; Beaumont repeated this lecture on March 27, 1854.
84. Beaumont, William, "Case of Traumatic Carotid Aneurism," *Braithwaite's Retrospect of Practical Medicine and Surgery*, 30 (January 1855), 130
85. Beaumont, William, "Case of Traumatic Carotid Aneurism," 130.
86. Beaumont, William, letter to Stratford, Samuel, February, 1854. Quoted in "Dr. Beaumont's Case of Aneurism," *Upper Canada Journal of Medical, Surgical and Physical Science*, 3 (1853–1854), 325–327.
87. Stratford, Samuel, "Rough Notes," 258.
88. *Report of an Investigation by the Trustees of the Toronto General Hospital into Certain Charges Against the Management of that Institution*(Toronto: Globe Book and Job Office, 22 King Street West, 1855).

89. Aikins, William Thomas, diary entry for January 13, 1856. Quoted in Godfrey, Charles, (1979), 77–78. Aikins' comments are useful, but they should be treated judiciously. In an 1854 diary entry, he says, for example, that the medical faculty at "Trinity is not failing but is gathering strength every day." This was just two years before its disintegration. See Spragge, George, (1966), 72.

90. Aikins, William Thomas, Diary entry for June 30, 1856. Quoted in Godfrey, Charles, (1979), 77. It is a pity that the crucial word in this text is illegible. Was Beaumont drunk, angry or simply sick? He had previously confessed at the Trustees' hearing that "I have often taken a glass of wine in the Hospital with some of the examining Board" (Report of an Investigation, 65), but being drunk on the job does seem rather out of character.

91. Clarke, Charles K., (1913).

92. Beaumont, William, "Clinical Lecture on a Deeply–Penetrating Wound of the Head, by a Rocket–Shaft passing through the left orbit," *Lancet* (June 14, 1862), 627.

93. Canniff, William, (1894), 263–267.

94. "The Death from Chloroform at the General Hospital," *The Daily Globe*, 20, #13 (Thursday, January 15, 1863), 3. "Important Medical Case: Inquiry into a Death from Chloroform," *The Daily Leader*, 10, #2,979 (Thursday, January 15, 1863), 3.

95. "The Use of Chloroform", *The Daily Globe*, 20, #14 (Friday, January 16, 1863), 3.

96. Britnell, W.E., ed., *County Marriage Registers of Ontario, Canada, 1858–1869*, 15(Toronto City) (Agincourt: Generation Press, 1986), 8; see also Ontario Genealogical Society, Toronto Branch, *Cathedral Church of St. James (Anglican) Marriages, 1800–1908*, p. 381 (fiche #4), record #4386, in St. James Anglican Cathedral Church Archives, 131 Adelaide Street East, Toronto, Ontario.

97. Sutherland, James, *City of Toronto Directory for 1867–8* (Toronto: W.C. Chewett, 1867), 147; "Rosedale Pioneer is Taken by Death," *Toronto Globe* 88, #25,396 (Monday, May 22, 1931), page 14; *St. James' Cemetery, Toronto: Register of Interments:* (May, 1931), "Charlotte Jarvis," Internment Number 47443, (Reel #1: January 1930–May, 1957), St. James' Anglican Cathedral Archives, 131 Adelaide Street East, Toronto, Ontario.

98. Canniff, William, "Experience among some of the Wounded who fell at the Battle of Limestone Ridge, June 2nd," *Canadian Medical Journal*, 2(1865–1866), 529–534.
99. Jack, Donald, (1981), 639.
100. Beaumont, William, "Cases of Stone in the Bladder — Lithotrity" *Canada Lancet*, 3, #1 (September, 1870), 35–37.
101. *Toronto Globe*, 32, #245 (whole number 7,979) (Wednesday, October 13, 1875), p. 2; *Toronto Globe*, 32, #246 (whole number 7,980) (Thursday, October 14, 1875), p. 2; *Toronto Mail*, 4, #1,108 (Wednesday, October 13, 1875), p. 1; *Toronto Mail*, 4, #1,109 (Thursday, October 14, 1875), p. 1.
102. Farnie, D.A., "The Textile Industry: Woven Fabrics", in Singer, Charles, Holmyard, E.J., Hall, A. Rupert, and Williams, Trevor, ed., *A History of Technology* vol. 5(Oxford: Clarendon Press, 1958), 569–574; see pages 589–590.
103. "Obituary — William Rawlins Beaumont, M.D., F.R.C.S. Eng", *British Medical Journal*, 2, (December 11, 1875), 750.

INDEX

Abernethy, John, 11, 17-9, 21, 35, 39.
Account of Some New Instruments..., 38.
Adelaide Street (Toronto), 99, 126, 143.
Aequanimitas (Osler), 136.
Aikins, William, 13, 65, 88, 101-2, 114, 116-122, 130, 133-4, 137, 154.
Aldersgate Street School, 18.
Amussat, Jean Zulema, 28-9.
Anatomical and Physiological Commentaries (Mayo), 21.
Anatomy and Surgical Treatment of Hernia (Cooper), 20-21.
Arabia, 32.
Army Medical Service, 36.
Arrowsmith, George, 148.
Atkinson, James, 77.
Augustinians, 16.
Austin Canons, 16.

Badgley, Francis, 95.
Bagot, Sir Charles, 50, 53, 58-9.
Baldwin, Robert, 53, 77, 86, 93-4.
Bank of Upper Canada, 48-50.
Barbados, 87, 95.
Barker, E.A.J., 145.
Barrett, Michael, 92.
Beard, G.L., 68.
Beaumont Court, 16.
Beaumont Street, 15, 33.
Beaumont, Ann (sister), 15.
Beaumont, Charlotte (daughter), 60, 101, 131-2, 140.
Beaumont, Charlotte (mother), 15-6.
Beaumont, Edward (brother), 15, 81, 101.
Beaumont, Edward (father), 15-6.
Beaumont, Herbert (son), 15, 101, 140, 142.
Beaumont, Mary Catherine (wife), 60, 101, 135.
Beer's Knife, 70, 72, 84.
Beer, George Joseph, 70.
Bell, Charles, 21.
Bell, Gary, 145-7, 149.
Berlin, 33, 86.
Berners Street, 33.
Bethune, Norman, 95.
Bethune, Professor, 133, 137, 139.
Blodgett, Shelburne C., 148, 150.
body-snatching, 64-65.
Bolding, John, 89.
Bonnycastle, Sir Richard, 48-9.

Booker, Colonel Alfred, 134.
Bovell, James, 57, 65, 87, 90, 95, 96, 100-1, 117, 129, 130, 136-7.
Braithwaite, W., 114.
Brent, J.W., 115-6.
British American Journal of Medical and Physical Sciences, 77, 96.
British Medical Journal, 142-3.
Brown, George, 81.
Brunel, 142-3.
Brunel, Isambard Kingdom, 143.
Brunel, Sir Marc Isambard, 143.
Buchanan, Charles William, 126.
Buller, John, 83-84.
Burns (Toronto General Hospital orderly), 115, 118.
Burnside Lying-In Department of the Toronto General Hospital, 52.
Burnside Lying-In Hospital, 64.
Burnside, Alexander, 49, 51, 52, 95

Calvin, John, 97.
Cambridge (University), 19, 39, 58, 63.
Cameron, Charles, 79.
Campobello, 134.
Canada Lancet, 136, 138, 142-3, 146-7.
Canada Medical and Surgical Journal, 142-3.
Canadas in 1841, 48-9.
Canadian Practitioner, 88.
Canniff Papers, 7.
Canniff, William, 13, 68, 69, 126, 133, 135, 139, 144, 154.
Cayley, William, 54.
Celsus, 122.
Chapman, Edward and William, 148, 152-3.
Charlton, M., 144.
cheiloplasty, 73.
Chevalier and Amici, 12.
chloroform, 12, 13, 129-131, 138, 154.
cholera, 51, 53, 55, 58, 67, 87, 111.
Christ's Hospital, 17.
Church of St. Mary's by the Bourne, 15.
Civil War (England), 17.
Civil War (United States), 134.
Clark, Edward, 150.
Clarke, Charles K., 123, 144.
Clarke, Edward, 87, 115.
Clarke, William, 34-35.
Clergy Reserves, 94, 107.

Clifford, James, 72-3.
Cobban, James, 82-3.
College of Physicians and Surgeons of Upper Canada, 51-2, 55, 103.
Connor, Skeffington, 104.
Cooper, Grace Rogers, 147.
Cooper, Sir Astley Paston, 20-1, 29, 87, G., 145.
Cosbie, W.G., 145.
Craigleigh (Toronto), 132.
Croft, Henry Holmes, 60, 61.
Cumberland, F.W., 104.
Colonist, 115, 118.

Daily Courant, 15.
Daily Globe, 80-1, 85, 96, 131.
Daly, Dominic, 77, 81.
Daviel's scoope, 71.
De Motu Cordis (Harvey), 16.
Deancroft (Toronto), 132.
Deazley, Thomas, 64.
Dennis, Colonel John Stoughton, 135.
Dickey, Benjamin, 78.
Dictionary of Canadian Biography, 6
Dieffenbach, Johann Friedrich, 33.
Dixon, James, 116.
Donnelly (Toronto General Hospital Nurse), 116, 118.
Dragoons, 14th, 50.
Draper, William Henry, 93.
Duffy, John, 82.
Duncan, John, 148, 152.
Durie, William, 49, 55, 57, 69.
eclectics, 139.

Edinburgh Royal Infirmary, 30.
Elgin, James Bruce, 102.
Elliott, Doctor, 135.
Encyclopedia Britannica, 145.
ether, 12, 129, 154.
Exostosis of Scapula (paper), 38.

Farrar, David, 86.
Farringdon Dispensary, 31.
Fawcett, Edward, 129-30.
Fawcett, Edward, 129.
Fenian Brotherhood, 134-5.
Fenian Raids, 134-5.
Fianna, 134.
Fidlar, Joshua, 86.
Fife, 55.
fistula instrument, 36-8, 146-7, 151, 153.
Fort Erie, 134-5.
Fraser, Doctor, 143-4, 152.
Fraser, John, 144.
Freeman, 147.
Fruin, Henry, 83.
Fulton, John, 139.

G., Thomas, 138.

Gardiner, 138.
Gardiner, J., 129.
Geikie, Doctor, 108, 137, 139.
Gerrard Street (Toronto), 10, 115, 121.
Gibbs, James, 17.
Gilchrist, John, 67.
Glenhurst (Toronto), 132, 140.
Godfrey, Charles, 145.
Good Doctors and Safe People (editorial), 119.
Graefe's forceps, 127.
Graefe, 127.
Grasset, Reverend, 132.
Great Fire of London, 17.
Gregory's Conspectus, 79.
Gunn, John, 76-7.
Guthrie, George James, 113.
Guy's Hospital, 20, 49, 61, 87.
Gwynne, William, 49-50, 53-4, 56, 59-61, 63-4, 67-9, 76-7, 86, 91, 93, 102.

Hagerman, 81.
Hahneman, Samuel, 139.
Hall, Cyrenius B., 137.
Hall, Marshall, 30.
Hallowell, William, 95, 130.
Hamilton, John, 77.
Hamilton, Joseph, 68-9, 75, 78.
Hampton, Doctor, 138.
Hanson, Henry, 76.
Harveian Orator, 144.
Harvey, John, 78, 81.
Harvey, William, 16.
Hastings, Horace Craft, 87.
Hawkins, Caesar, 72.
Henwood, Edwin, 76, 87.
Henwood, Reginald, 76-7.
Hermann, H., 37.
hernia, 21, 34, 35.
Herod, George Samuel, 79, 81.
Herrick, George, 49, 56-7, 60, 65, 67-9, 75, 77-8, 101-2, 104, 116-7.
Hincks Act, 57, 107, 136.
Hincks, Sir Francis, 107, 108.
Hipkins, Edward, 86.
Hippocrates, 37, 122, 136, 152.
History of the Toronto General Hospital (Clarke), 144.
Hodder, 10, 57, 63-5, 87, 90, 95-6, 99, 100, 114, 116-7, 124, 129-30, 133, 135-9, 142.
Holmes, George, 86.
homeopathy, 139.
Hornby, Robert, 49, 55-7, 67-9, 78, 86.
Hospital for Sick Children (Toronto), 143.
Hospital Street (Toronto), 54.
Hotham, Sir Beaumont, 16.
Howe, Elias, 148-153.
Humphreys, Mrs., 129-30.

Humphreys, Richard, 129-131.
Hunt, Walter, 148-150, 152-3.
Hunter, Robert, 76, 80-1, 85-6, 88.
Invention of the Sewing Machine (article), 147.

iris forceps, 11, 71, 126-129, 151.
Islington Dispensary, 33-4.

Jack, Donald, 13.
Jarvis, Edgar Beaumont, 131-2.
Jarvis, Edgar John, 131-2, 140.
Jarvis, Frederick Starr, 131.
Jarvis, Herbert Cherriman, 140.
Jarvis, Louis Raymond, 140.
Jarvis, Paul, 132.
Jarvis, Susan Isabella, 131.
Jefferson Medical Colege, 88.
Johns Hopkins University, 136.
Johnson, Arthur Jukes, 123-4.
Johnson, William, 136.
Jugandi, Michelle, 7.

King Edward VII Hospital for Officers, 16.
King George IV, 21.
King's College, 6, 8, 13, 28, 49-64, 67, 69, 75-6, 78-9, 81, 87, 90-5, 107, 137, 144, 154.
King, Hugh, 89.
King, John, 49, 52-4, 56-7, 65, 68-9, 75, 129.
Krems, Balthasar, 148-9, 153.

Lancet, 18, 30, 113-4, 122, 126, 128, 145-7, 150-2.
Langenbeck, 127.
Langstaff, 101.
Lawlor, Michael, 129.
Lawrence, Sir William, 21, 28, 37, 71-2, 147.
Learned, Arthur, 12.
Lennon, John (medical student), 116.
Lewton, Frederick A., 147.
Li, Alison, 7.
Lister, Joseph, 13.
Liston, Robert, 12, 39.
lithotomy, 121-2, 138, 154.
lithotrity, 138-9.
Lizars, John Lizars, 133.
London Infirmary for Curing Diseases of the Eye, 21.
London International Exhibition, 12.
London Medical and Physical Journal, 32.
London Medical Gazette, 33, 35-6, 38, 71, 146.
Long, Crawford Williamson, 12.
Long, Michael George, 76.
Lord, Henry, 78.

Lot Street, 49, 56, 62, 64.
Lunatic Asylum, 50, 52-3, 57, 65, 98.
Lying-In Hospital, 51-2, 64, 98.
Lyons, William, 66.

Macaulay Town (York), 63.
Macdonald, John A., 94, 97.
Macdonnell, Bishop Alexander, 93.
Mackenzie Rebellion, 63.
Macklem, Thomas Clark, 75.
Magendie, François, 21.
Marshall, Mary Ann, 73-4.
Marshall, N., 104.
Maternity Lying-In Hospital and General Dispensary, 99.
Maunoir's scissors, 70-1, 83-4.
Mayo, Herbert, 21.
McCaul, John, 60, 92.
McDougall, Alexander, 79.
McGill College (Montreal), 55, 75.
McGill University, (Montreal), 136, 142.
McGregor, James, 36, 39.
McHugh, James, 99-100.
McIlmurray, James, 49, 54, 56.
McKennzie's Weekly Message, 107.
McNicholas, John, 84-5.
Medical Board, 50-8, 66-9, 75-81, 85-6, 88, 90, 99, 102-3, 108, 119, 144, 154.
Medical Gazette, 33, 35-6, 38, 71, 146.
Medical Profession in Upper Canada (Canniff), 144.
Medicine for Ontario (Godfrey), 145.
Medico-Chirurgical and Ethical Society, 124.
Medico-Chirurgical Review, 33
Medico-Chirurgical Society, 77
Medico-Chirurgical Transactions, 99, 128, 151.
Melville, Henry, 95-6, 100.
Meredith, Allen, 81.
Merigold, 131.
Methodists, 93, 107.
Middlesex Hospital, 21.
Morrison, 101.
Moss Hall (Toronto), 137.
Mr. A., 82-3.
Murray, Sir George, 59.

National School of Upper Canada, 49.
Neilsen, John B., 2
Nichol, James, 78.
Nichols, Richard, 122-3.
Nicol, William Bulmer, 58, 60, 68-9, 75-6, 78.
nitrous oxide, 154.
Northumberland Battalion, 58.

O'Brien, Colonel Edward George, 53.
O'Brien, Lucius, 49, 53-5, 57, 96.

187

O'Brien, William Smith, 10.
O'Mahoney, John, 134.
O'Neill, John, 134.
Ogden, C.R., 79.
Ogden, Uzziel, 88, 117, 154.
Ogden, William Winslow, 65.
Ontario College of Physicians and Sorgeons, 88.
Ontario Medical Act, 139.
Ontario Medical Association, 62.
opium, 71, 83-4, 100.
Orr, Joseph, 49, 53, 56.
Osgoode Hall, 49.
Osler, William, 12-3, 87, 136, 154-5.

Paget, Sir James, 18-9, 21, 33-34, 37, 143-4, 146-7, 152.
Paris Academy of Medicine, 28.
Park, George Hamilton, 63.
Pasteur, 13.
Paterson, G.R., 2
Perry, Egerton, 87.
Peter Street (Toronto), 61, 98.
Pharmocopoeia Londinensis, 79.
Phelan, John, 86.
Phelpes, Orson C., 149-50.
Pilon, Henri, 6.
Plarr's Lives of the Fellows of the Royal College of Surgeons, 144, 145.
Plymouth Royal Marine Hospital, 86.
Port Colborne, Ontario, 134-5.
Pott, Percival, 17.
Potter, Richard, 60.
Powell, Newton Albert, 145.
Power, D'Arcy, 37, 145-6.
Practical Lithotomy and Lithotrity, 138.
Presbyterians, 107.
Proceedings of the Royal Medical and Chirurgical Society, 144.
Provincial Lying-In Hospital and Vaccine Institute, 99.

Quebec, 2, 52-4, 78.
Queen Victoria, 34, 96.
Queen's College, Kingston, 93.
Queenston Heights, 68.
Queenston, 63.

Rahere, 16.
Rebellion of 1837, 39, 51, 54, 58-9, 63.
Rees, William, 49, 52-7.
Regiopolis College, Kingston, 93.
Reid, John (doctor), 78.
Reid, John (patient), 38-9.
Retrospect of Practical Medicine and Surgery, 114, 122.
Richardson, James, 13, 61-2, 101, 118, 137, 154.
Roberts, Colonel William, 134.

Roberts, David, 6.
Rolph School, 55, 63-4, 69, 76, 88, 92, 98-9, 103, 107, 115-6, 119, 136-7, 139, 154.
Rolph, John, 51, 55, 57, 61-4, 65, 101-3, 107-8, 119, 137.
Roman Catholic Orphan Asylum, 99.
Rossin House, 10.
Royal Artillery, 55.
Royal College of Surgeons of England, 17, 20, 29-32, 37-9, 49, 51, 54, 61-4, 68, 78, 86, 126, 143-5, 147.
Royal College of Physicians (London), 39.
Royal Engineers, 48.
Royal Foresters, 51.
Royal Medical and Chirurgical Society, 38-9, 71-2, 128, 144.
Rule Number Five, 96.
Russell, Gavin, 78.
Ryall, Doctor, 135.

Saint, Thomas, 148, 152.
Salmon, James Moon, 78.
Salpêtrière Hospital, 28.
Sandor, Monica, 6.
Scadding, Henry, 60.
Scarpa's needle, 71, 84, 89.
Schmutter, Godfrey H., 86.
Scott, John, 49, 57, 98.
Scott, William, 86.
Scott, William, 86.
Seager, Samuel, 79.
Semi-Weekly Leader, 110-1.
Servant in the House (article), 147.
Sewell, S.E., 79.
Shakespeare Tavern, 10, 125.
Shea, Hannah, 74.
Simeonites, 19.
Simpson, James Young, 12, 129.
Simpson, Robert, 89-90.
Sims, James Marion, 12.
Singer Sewing Machine, 3, 11, 142-4, 145, 147-153.
Singer, Isaac Merritt, 145, 147-154.
Smithsonian Institution, 147.
Société Universelle d'Opthalmologie, 128.
Spear, Robert, 39.
Spragge, George W., 145.
St. Bartholomew's Hospital, 16-21, 31, 33-4, 37, 63, 122, 143.
St. James Cathedral (Toronto), 6, 60, 101, 131-2.
St. Marylebone (London), 15.
St. Patrick's Society, 54.
St. Thomas's Hospital, 20, 49.
Stephens, James, 134.
Sterves, 112-3.
Stone, T.M., 143-4, 152.

Stone, Thomas Arthur, 144.
Strachan, John, 7, 50, 55, 59, 60, 63, 85, 94-5, 137.
Stratford, Samuel John, 98, 100, 109, 112-5, 118, 122, .
Stricture of the Urethra, 138.
Strother, Joshua, 69-71.
Sullivan, Henry, 49, 51, 60-2, 67, 68-9, 76-7, 86, .
Sullivan, Robert Baldwin, 51.
Sweeney, General, 134.
Sylvan Tower (Toronto), 132.

T., William, 138.
Telfer, Walter, 49, 54, 55, 57, 65, 67-9, 75, 102, 117.
Temple, James Algernon, 142.
Thimonnier, Barthelemy, 148, 153.
Thirty Nine Articles, 59, 96.
Thirty-Sixth Canon, 96.
Thomas, John S., 67.
Thompson, Sir Henry, 138.
Thomson, Samuel, 139.
Tiemann, George, 143, 147, 151.
Toronto Academy of Medicine, 37, 39, 145.
Toronto, Bulletin of the Academy of Medicine, 145.
Toronto Colonist, 115, 118.
Toronto Dispensary, 143.
Toronto Eye Infirmary, 98, 100.
Toronto General Dispensary and Lying-In Hospital, 98.
Toronto Globe, 80-1, 85, 96, 131.
Toronto Hospital/Toronto General Hospital, 7, 10, 39, 50, 52, 54-6, 62, 64, 68-9, 75, 82, 84, 87-9, 92, 98-9, 102, 104, 108-12, 115-24, 127, 129-32, 138, 144-6, 154. 96, 100, 102, 112, 115, 128, 138, 144,
Toronto Hospital Board, 50, 120.
Toronto Mechanics' Institute, 103, 139.
Toronto Patriot, 95.
Torsion of Arteries (Amussat), 28.
Townsend, P.S., 143.
trichina spiralis, 34.
Trinity College, 6, 8, 52, 63, 65, 87, 96, 98, 108, 136-7, 139, 142, 144-5.
Trinity College, Dublin, 52-3.
Trinity Medical College (article), 144.
Turner, John, 19-20.
typhus, 68.

University Bill, 53, 93-4, 104.
University College, 107.
University of Brussels, 29.
University of Edinburgh, 20, 30, 52-3, 55-7, 63, 68, 75-6, 87, 95, 133.
University of New York, 76, 145.
University of Pennsylvania, 136.

University of Toronto, 6, 13, 58, 65, 88, 94, 97-9, 103-4, 107-8, 118-9, 136-7, 154.
University of Trinity College, 52.
Upper Canada Journal of Medical Surgical and Physical Science, 64, 71, 73, 87, 96, 100, 103, 109, 113-4.
Upper Canada Academy (Cobourg), 93.
Upper Canada Bank, 48-50.
Upper Canada College, 49, 91-2.
Upper Canada School of Medicine, 63, 95, 98.

Vaccine Institute, 54, 99.
vaginal speculum, 11-2, 36-8, 146-7, 152-3.
Valsalva's Method, 112-3.
Veritas (anonymous letter), 116.
Victoria College, 6, 88, 107, 133, 137.
Virchow, Rudolf, 34.

Wakley, Thomas, 18, 30,
Wallace, Joseph, 70-1.
Wallace, William Stewart, 108.
Warren, J.W., 102.
Wasbrick, John Clark, 87.
Watkins, James, 10, 11, 125-6.
Weisenthal, Charles E., 148-9.
Weiss, 138.
Wells, Horace, 12.
Wells, Sir Thomas Spencer, 12.
Welton, Thurston Scott, 144.
Wesley, John, 97.
West York Regiment, 52.
Widmer, Christopher 49-56, 59-60, 66-9, 75, 78, 98-104, 112, 114, 116, 118, 119, 122-5, 132.
Wilson, William H., 86.
Woolbank, Samuel Sedden, 87.
Workman, Joseph, 49, 55, 63, 101-3, 137.
Wright, Henry Case, 87.
Wright, Henry Hover, 119.

Yonge Street, 6, 51, 53-5, 144.
York Volunteers, 54.
Yorkville (Toronto), 132, 140.

Zieber, George, 150.
Zimmermann, Richard, 142.